The BioChemical Machine

The
BioChemical Machine

Empowering Your Body Chemistry

Eleonora De Lennart

BIG APPLE VISION BOOKS
An Imprint of Big Apple Vision Publishers

The information in this book is based on the latest scientific research. However, the author and publisher are not prescribing and assume no responsibility. However, in no way should this information be considered a substitute for competent health care by the professional of your choice. In the event you use this information without your doctor's approval, you are prescribing for yourself, which is your constitutional right.

BIG APPLE VISION BOOKS
An Imprint of Big Apple Vision Publishers, New York

Library of Congress Cataloging-in-Publication Data

Copyright © 1996, 1999, 2000, 2003 by Eleonora De Lennart
ISBN: 0-9724327-0-1
www.BigAppleVision.com

Second printing,: May 2004

Big Apple Vision® is a registered trademark of Big Apple Vision Publishing, Inc.

Printed in Canada

Cover designed by George Foster

ACKNOWLEDGMENTS

Without courageous scientists like Professor Luke Burke, Professor Claus Leitzmann, Professor Julian Jaynes, Professor Helmut Minne, Professor Joachim Seidl, Dr. Ernest Obie, Dr. Quazi Al Tariq, M.D., Dr. Stephen Chukumba, Sharon Y. Robinson, Beatrice Ymiama, M.D., James C. Romano, M.D.; inspirations like Linda Fite and Herb Trimpe, Michael Weinstein and Adrienne Heald; friends like Michael R. Wehr; and Moira Joyce; attorneys like Rebecca Millouras Lettre, Michael Graff and family like my husband (who shares my belief in the importance of fighting for the future of humankind), my great mother (who taught me how to fight), and the greatest sister in the world—a book like The BioChemical Machine *wouldn't have come to life.*

Contents

Foreword

By Dr. Quazi Al Tariq, Horton Hospital (affiliate of New York Presbyterian Hospital); Arden Hill Hospital; Mid-Hudson Forensic Psych. Center; Goshen Residential Center

"In yourself has to burn, what you want to light in other people" (Augustinus). This sentence came into my mind when I spoke to Eleonora De Lennart and read her scientifically sound research. Though the content of the book is scientific, it is entertaining, thrilling, and understandable for every layperson. I am impressed by De Lennart's findings and further development of a significant research.

In this book you will learn and understand the truth about dangerous diets, the importance of fat, the truth about cholesterol, and how to eat your food chemically perfect—the easy way. It is a well-known myth that fat is bad for health. However, while reading this book, you will be surprised to learn the harsh truth about fat—that it is an integral part of our body. Without it, life is impossible. This is backed by numerous scientific researches.

It's all about chemical imbalances within the body. These imbalances lead to multiple health problems including heart disease, cancer, hyperlipidemia, and most notably obesity. However, by eating according to the perfect match of food chemistry and body chemistry you will get total control over your health and its side effect: weight problems. By showing the history of our eating habits, De Lennart makes the logic of the research very clear. The A&B is a scientific way of eating that embraces all types of food from the rich offering of our modern world.

The *BioChemical Machine* is truly a comprehensive, easy to read guide for the whole family. This book is recommended for both the general reader and professionals. It is for healthy people who care for prevention and for sick people. Those who are ill will have a realistic chance to "repair" their BioChemical Machine in order to be able to look forward to a longer and happier life without pain.

It is a wonderful resource for healthy meal planning. It tackles most of the nutritional issues that concerns Americans today. No matter what your age, you will find it useful and easy to understand. Beliefs about eating are changing. The focus has moved from dieting and losing weight to establishing healthful overall eating habits to help one feel good, live healthy, and prevent disease.

This book focuses on all areas of one's concern—diet, nutrition and diseases. The research is scientifically sound. This is a must-read book for every household.

Quazi Al Tariq, M.D.

Introduction

IN THE NAME OF SCIENCE

Although he is not a clergyman, I believe Luke Burke, PhD, a professor at Rutgers University in New Jersey, will one day be seen as saint to millions of Americans. Currently chairman of the Department of Chemistry, Doctor Burke played an instrumental role in a revolutionary discovery that I believe will provide millions of people with the necessary information for solving their most challenging health and weight problems.

Prior to my first meeting with Professor Burke, I was made aware of his demanding reputation by Sharon Robinson. A senior chemist at the New Jersey Department of Health, Robinson had come to realize that my work had the potential to help millions of people. However, before I presented Professor Burke with my research that clarified and expanded on the acid-alkaline balance research of William Howard Hay for his critique, she warned me about her mentor: "Nothing unscientific! No imperfections!"

1

Up to this point, I had not yet made the groundbreaking discovery of the concept of the "good," "bad," and "extreme-bad" proteins, which, as you will realize while reading the book, is the root of many if not all the health and weight evils of our modern times. Like many of the "diet gurus," whose theories I scorned, I was stuck with the tired and unscientific message of "separating carbohydrates and proteins." And yes, even though I had already completed the original A&B Chart, it was still not the revolutionary match of food chemistry and body chemistry that you will find on the A&B Charts included in this book.

But before I share my most important* discoveries with you—discoveries which I believe have the potential to alter weight and health problems forever—I would like to tell you why I got involved with something that wasn't even connected to my field of expertise. My specialty is the Science of Consciousness and my major research, which has been endorsed by renowned scientists, is *The Race That Should Be Human*. I am not a "medicine-man" or biochemist. And yet, it was my personal experience and research—done first and foremost for my family (who patiently served as first guinea pigs and test persons) and for myself—that ultimately led to the decision to write *The BioChemical Machine*.

---

*I say "most important," because of "the trillions of dollars for health-care costs in a world that quadrupled in population in one century…and it's heading for 9 to 10 billion." Time, November 1, 1999, page 87

"In the year 2021, every American will be overweight. Health care costs…will reach $16 trillion by the year 2020." American Heart Association, 9/1998.

Yes, there were many moments when I deeply regretted ever having touched this project. I had no idea what I was getting myself into or what I was putting at risk. But ultimately, I am happy that I did what I had to do because it has already positively impacted so many lives, including those of my husband, my sisters, my mother, my mother-in-law and yes, my own. Beyond that, it made life worth living! A life without pain, ailments, fatigue, and a life where there is no daily struggle with something we all love to do, namely, eating.

My Personal Journey

Twenty years ago, I began a journey that I am convinced saved my life. In my early 20s, I was in great shape, energetic and slim. But as I grew older, I began to struggle with a variety of health problems. I was plagued by fatigue and pain caused by what I would later learn to be self-poisoning. I suffered through a litany of ailments, from liver, pancreas, and kidney diseases to diabetes, tumors, fatigue, and clinical depression. Making matters worse, I struggled with my weight and the associated frustrations of ineffective diets and useless "magic" pills.

I didn't realize that I was already caught up in the most vicious and telltale cycles of our very existence: pathological fatigue. This is the first sign that something is wrong with the balance of the body chemistry. And I certainly didn't know that the causes of fatigue are closely related to the causes of disease. As I would learn, pathological fatigue is the result of unknowingly poisoning oneself through chemically wrong eating.

3

Furthermore, increasing weight problems, and the subsequent involvement with alleged "miracle diets," took their toll. Like many others confronted with similar health ailments, I bought into false claims that did nothing more than complicate my problems.

Finally, in the summer of 1983, I hit a low point in my life. I was experiencing pain in every fiber of my body and was so weak that I could hardly walk. It was late in the evening and I remember thinking I needed professional help and I needed it fast. But, because of the hour, I could not contact my regular physician. In retrospect, this turned out to be a blessing in disguise because it led me to call my friend John, a specialist in internal medicine. He was one of those incredibly dedicated professionals who attend every key seminar around the country that focuses on the latest medical research. I was hopeful he would be able to offer me something new. Perhaps a miracle pill or at least information on the latest revolutionary medical procedure or treatment.

Instead, he introduced me to a way of approaching food that would change my life forever. After examining my once energetic body, he asked about my eating habits. Then, instead of prescribing medication, which I expected, he pulled a little book from his pocket, *A New Health Era* by William Howard Hay, M.D.[1] He explained that the cause of my fatigue and body pains could be directly attributed to an imbalance in my body chemistry. The book, he said, outlined a method of learning to live with food in a way that would bring my body chemistry back into alignment. I was surprised, and admittedly, *very* disappointed.

4

Not only had I never heard of this Dr. Hay, I had no interest in trying any more diet programs.

But John stressed that this was not a diet. "It's a scientifically documented method for smart eating," he said. "It's about your body chemistry and serves as both prevention and cure...as a side effect, your weight will take care of itself."

I had heard this promise before. I couldn't imagine that something as ordinary as food could be the solution to my health and weight problems. Yet, I knew I could trust John and above all, I felt so ill, that I decided to follow his instructions even though I was sure they would fail.

Dr. William Hay

Dr. William Howard Hay graduated from New York University on March 26, 1891, and practiced medicine and general surgery (see appendix). Many of his original guidelines are still employed by nutritionists and dieticians. His focus was the acid-alkaline balance and his advice was simple: eat what nature offers. In Dr. Hay's day, his approach was sound since life (and food) was still pretty simple. There were no fast food restaurants and no super size supermarkets with unimaginable numbers of delicious and mouthwatering products. Instead, we shopped at Ma & Pa shops like the neighborhood butcher and other small stores. Smaller incomes and simpler times meant less availability of the types of foods that are so damaging to our BioChemical Machine.

Be that as it may, that very night I didn't think about bygone times; I just did as John suggested. I changed my eating habits and almost immediately began feeling better. It was almost like the cartoon figure Popeye, who, after eating his spinach, experiences an immediate reaction. After a few days, my energy began to return and, slowly but surely, the strange pains in my body began to lessen. I was stunned and didn't know what to make of it. But I stuck to the method religiously. I lost 25 pounds in six weeks and slowly began overcoming the other health problems that had plagued me for so long. As long as I ate properly—choosing foods based on their chemical compatibility—I continued to make progress. It didn't matter if I ate baked potatoes with butter, wheat bread with mayonnaise, or pizza with olives, the program worked! *Little did I know at the time, the best was yet to come.*

As I moved into my 40s, my life was better than ever. Unfortunately, I was unaware that there was a new horror lurking around the corner that would plague my life with 24-hour pain, rheumatoid arthritis. As the illness progressed, my thumb became crippled and the pain in my bones, especially my hipbones, increased dramatically. I needed a cane to get up from the couch. Despite heavy painkillers, the pain didn't stop. Finding no relief from traditional treatments, I started to research the illness. I couldn't understand why this was happening to my body after eating correctly for so long.

For many years, I had avoided drinking milk because of its pesticides, chemicals, and hormones. I have no doubt that eliminating it from my diet played a big part in my body's calcium deficiency.

But the more I researched, the more I realized that this was not the whole cause of my affliction. If it was, all arthritic and osteoarthritic cases could be cured by drinking more milk and eating more dairy products. Unfortunately, it's not that simple.

In retrospect, it was the key experience of my rheumatoid arthritis (or rather my panic over seeing my crippled thumb and imagining this happening to the rest of my body) that led to my most important and landmark discovery—**the vast chemical differences between "good" and "bad" proteins—and their impact on the health of our biochemical machine**. Knowing the distinction between "good" and "bad" proteins and understanding how to counteract their impact on your overall health and weight will empower you to control your body's vitality.

The very foundation of the A&B Method is built upon my groundbreaking research of "good" and "bad" proteins—and the protein deficiency mostly caused by high protein/low carb diets, which sounds paradoxical, but, as my research proves, is not. With the A&B Method you can eat everything from potatoes and pizza to pasta, rice, chocolate, wheat bread, bananas, beer and wine without gaining weight—but improving health and energy.

At this point I would like to mention that it seems some of the diet gurus have read the European edition of my book — copyright 1996. Obviously, they found my research inspiring. Because, besides "borrowing" from my concepts, they mistakenly invented the idea of good and bad carbohydrates. **THIS IS NONSENSE**. There is no such thing as bad carbohydrates.

It is common knowledge that some carbohydrates are less healthy than others, but NEVER as hazardous as the "bad" and "extreme-bad" proteins central to many of today's popular high protein/low carb diets. Carbohydrates are essential for your well-being—because carbohydrates (besides fat) are the number one and two suppliers of energy. **AGAIN, I EMPHASIZE** with the A&B Method you can eat everything from potatoes and pizza to pasta, rice, chocolate, wheat bread, bananas, beer and wine without gaining weight—but gaining health and energy.

Having experienced the positive impact of Hay's work, I wondered why everyone didn't know about it. When I looked closer, I found the answer. As a result of his research on the acid-alkaline balance and alkaline reserve, Hay had concluded that the root of all physical (and psychological) evil is directly related to the body's chemical imbalance. "All forms of disease and weight problems fall under one heading—chemical imbalance."[2]

Such revolutionary investigations and discoveries have been known to lead to a Nobel Prize. But that wasn't the case here. On the contrary, the scientific community dismissed his groundbreaking research!

As I would soon discover, there was an obstacle that allowed the quacks to distort Hay's work. Although his revolutionary research was primarily about acid-alkaline balance, he simplified part of the food chemistry findings and spoke of "separating carbohydrates from proteins."

This was his biggest mistake. Simply put, it was unscientific. Almost every food item consists of proteins and carbohydrates at the same time. Yet, even if his conclusions were partially wrong, his basic premise was still sound. For the scientific community, however, results must be perfect, which was not the case with Dr. Hay's findings.

Therefore, until recently we had missed out on the benefits of his research. I truly believe Hay's findings were largely responsible for saving my life. I also believe that the combination of Hay's work and my expansion of his basic research can benefit millions of people, not only in terms of prevention, but also to escape the vicious cycle of gurus and their never-ending miracle diets. I am living proof of the program's success, as are so many others. Everyone I convinced to try the A&B Method has succeeded. Ultimately, it was the program's simple success, and not the need for scientific proof, that served as my driving force.

However, I knew it was proof that would ultimately return Hay's reputation to good standing in the scientific community. Dr. Hay didn't involve food chemists in his work, as he should have, and he oversimplified terms to enable ordinary people to profit from his research. That was good thinking, but, and here is the big but, at the same time he created a loophole for those who would make billions of dollars by shamelessly using portions (especially the wrong ones!) of his findings. Gurus shaped his research into hazardous, ill-advised diets. Forty years after his death, Hay was dismissed as a quack. He became the father of all food-combining gurus, diet du jour starlets, and nutritionist wannabes. Whoever speaks of "food-combining diets" or "combination diets" or urges you to omit certain food groups distorts Dr. Hay's beneficial research. Unwittingly, despite his good intentions, Dr. Hay—the originator of scientific eating—had inspired money-hungry people to turn the BioChemical Machine into a money making machine.

Dr. Hay's findings about the acid-alkaline balance and the vital alkaline reserve should be considered a major research finding. Unfortunately, Dr. Hay had come up with the right idea at the wrong time; a time when the pharmaceutical industry was on the rise, and the focus was on cure, not prevention or side effects. Propaganda hammered miracle drugs into our parents' minds until they and the following generations believed that a pill could do anything. But we know this is just not true. My desire to clarify the misconceptions about Dr. Hay's research—and bring his findings to light—grew into a driving passion. Above all, I wanted to clear his reputation within the scientific community.

And so, with a lot of conviction and after a lot of hard work (that included developing the A&B Chart in conjunction with food chemists), I did what I had to do as the first step to restoring Dr. Hay's good name: I reached out to the scientific community. As I said, Sharon Robinson of the New Jersey Department of Health, introduced me to Dr. Burke, and warned me of his intractability when it came to scientific facts. But, since I was about to resurrect seriously significant research, I decided that Luke Burke was the right person to contact.

In the summer of 1997, I called Professor Burke, sent him my work, and arranged an appointment. When I entered his modern office for the first time, he was very kind, no question about it. He was much taller, younger, and sportier than I'd expected, but precisely as sharp as one would expect of such a highly respected scientist. I felt that he didn't really know what to think of me. Here I was, full of passion to help humankind, anxiously awaiting his reaction to my work. On top of his desk sat my open manuscript. He looked at the book as if to confirm he had received something so unscientific from me. After all, high-profile professors from Princeton University, Munich University, New Jersey State College, Denver University, and Hagia Academy had endorsed my major research dealing with societal problems and the science of consciousness, *The Race That Should Be Human.*

"Do you *really* believe that separating carbohydrates from proteins is the solution for health and weight problems? That's nonsense! I can't associate my name with something unscientific like that," he thundered.

Obviously, he had already made up his mind. I knew that if I couldn't convince this hard-evidence-oriented scientist, Dr. Hay's research would always remain in the dim zone of quacks. I told Professor Burke that I truly believed I would be dead if I had not found and used this program over the past 15 years. I related my litany of surgeries and the agony of trying every diet from high-protein to pills. I presented him with test results gathered by the German physician Dr. Ludwig Walb, one of the doctors who attempted to prove Dr. Hay right. These publications didn't impress him at all. "If this were serious research," Professor Burke said, "I would have received it directly from the scientists or the institutions themselves.

That's the usual procedure." To demonstrate, he showed me a letter from other German researchers, which he had received that very same day, as well as some papers from the Max Planck Institute in Germany.

"But perhaps they didn't understand how it works?" I said, trying to defend Dr. Walb's good intentions to spread Dr. Hay's teachings. I sensed that an invisible wall surrounded Professor Burke, separating him from my passion. I realized that I was defending myself while fighting for the truth; for something that I believed with all my heart. I realized that it was most likely the endorsement of Professor Julian Jaynes of Princeton University or the book's title that explained why Professor Burke decided to meet with me in the first place. I know the title of the book had caught his attention. He very much liked my idea of comparing the body to a BioChemical Machine. Despite his skepticism, there was something about my work that held his attention.

All of a sudden, he interrupted my thoughts and asked: "Why are you doing this project?"

"Because I'm so angry," I said and pointed to his computer, which in a moment of frustration, I confused with a television. I explained to him that the misleading ads on TV were making me angry, but I was especially angry with medical doctors who used their image to sell dangerous diets in order to make millions of dollars, often without regard for people's lives.* "More than 100,000 Americans will die this year alone due to improper eating habits,"[3]

---

*Those who promote diet products, slimming drinks and diet pills contribute to a $32 billion dollar industry.

I said, "Most people don't understand that heartburn is the first sign of chronic disease in the making. They don't realize that fatigue, illness and obesity are all intertwined. Americans are increasingly overweight, and we must do something about escalating health-care costs. It's as important as solving our environmental problems. It's as important as solving our political problems. It's about future generations. It's about changing minds, and it's also about health consciousness."

I went on to tell him about my research and my conviction to contribute whatever I could to help solve the problems of this dramatically changing world in this new millennium. "Everyone who learns to balance his or her own body chemistry will profit from it and will have the same energy as I have today," I told him.

"How can you prove what you say?" he said.

"I am the living proof!" I said.

"But that's not scientific," he said, smashing my explanations. Gotcha!

And so, with all my remaining energy, I tried one more time to convince the man whom I hoped would help me get this research into the right hands at American universities, and ultimately, the scientific community. "I found a cure for arthritis!" I suddenly said. "I developed a milk and apple therapy, a natural miracle drug!" And I added, "You probably don't know what it means to be in pain day in and day out." I was determined that I wouldn't leave his office until I had convinced him to introduce me to other scientists. This was my goal.

I told him about people who had profited from the A&B Method, people who at one time could not walk or live without painkillers. I spoke of my mother-in-law, who had been scheduled for surgery, but canceled the procedure due to her remarkable recovery; and I told him about my dentist's husband, who was scheduled for hip surgery and, after two weeks of following the A&B Method, came dancing to my house.

"They have medical records in black and white!" I told Professor Burke. "I myself needed a cane to get up from a chair before I began this method of eating." Burke looked at me, trying to figure out whether I was telling the truth, since I walk like a young girl.

"This program works. I know that the theory of separating carbohydrates from proteins is an over-simplification of great research, but I also know there is something here," I told Professor Burke.

He looked into my eyes and said, "Well, then, go and find it and than come back."

During the following weeks, I worked feverishly polishing my research. When I walked with my beloved German shepherd, Quinky, I had only one question on my mind: what is behind the theory of separating proteins from carbohydrates? It was during a follow-up meeting with Professor Burke that he came up with something I had not immediately recognized as revolutionary.

"The A&B principles are very interesting," he said, referring to my A&B Chart. "You don't separate the proteins from the carbohydrates."

I looked at him, speechless. This was the missing link!

On my return trip home, my mind was completely occupied with Professor Burke's words. Once home, I stormed into my office, ignoring the joyful greetings of my dog, to review the A&B Chart. Burke was right! On the chart, I had not separated carbohydrates from proteins. According to their chemistry, I had put vegetables into three groups, fruits in three, meat in two, fish in two, dairy products in two, nuts in two, and even eggs into two groups. Carbohydrates themselves were divided into three groups. In addition, I had an additional group, the Neutrals, which included selected dairy, meat, and fish products that, according to most diet gurus, should not be eaten with carbohydrates, vegetables, fruits, and nuts.

This was it! By trial and error I had discovered sound scientific principles to support the A&B Method.

This perfect match of food chemistry and body chemistry maintains the vital alkaline buffer that supports the proper balance of acid and alkalinity in the blood, which in turn prevents us from poisoning ourselves. At that moment, it became clear to me that this omission was the primary reason Dr. Hay never received his Nobel Prize. Now, instead of looking solely toward genetic engineering and other expensive interference with our BioChemical Machine, we can employ the simplest and most satisfying thing in the world—food—to dramatically improve our health.

Initially, it was Professor Burke's intractability that challenged me to further develop Dr. Hay's findings. Soon after, my completed research was to receive support from eminent authorities such as Professor Helmut Minne,* Dr. Quazi Al Tariq,** Professor Claus Leitzmann,*** Dr. Beatrice Inyama, and Dr. Ernest Obie. These respected members of the scientific and medical establishment had originally refused to endorse Dr. Hay's research.

Professor Minne had even called it "hocus-pocus." Today, Minne and others enthusiastically endorse and support my work.

Patients of other physicians**** have benefited from the A&B Method to alleviate the effects of such conditions like diabetes, obesity, heart disease, cancer, kidney disease, arteriosclerosis, arthritis, osteoporosis, rheumatism, allergies, cholesterol problems, ulcers, even multiple sclerosis (in combination with electro-neural-therapy, acc. to Croon*****).

Now, so can you.

The A&B Method will not interfere with MEDICAL TREATMENTS. On the contrary, this program is designed to ENHANCE its EFFECTIVENESS. As with any new program, first consult with your physician before starting the A&B Method.

---

*Professor Helmut Minne, University of Heidelberg, Chairman of the Board of Directors of the Kuratorium Knochengesundheit [bone health], e.V./Clinic Der Fuerstenhof, Bad Pyrmont.

**Dr. Quazi Al-Tariq, M.D., Horton Hospital (affiliate of New York Presbyterian), Arden Hill Hospital, Mid Hudson Forensic Psyc. Center, Goshen Residential Center.

***Professor Claus Leitzmann, Justus Liebig University; author of about 500 publications and books in the field of Nutrition Science. Among them, the "Dictionary of Nutrition," translated into English, French, Italian and Spanish (Ulmer).

****Dr. Ragnar Berg,[4] the chemist, Fred W. Koch, Dr. Friedrich Sander,[5] Professor Louis-Claude Vincent, Dr. Berthold Kern, Dr. Michael Worlitschek, Dr. Eduard A. Brecht[6] Dr. Hermann Aihara,[7] Professor Lothar Wendt, Dr. Bircher-Brenner,[8] Professor W. Zabel, Dr. Ludwig Walb.

*****Physicians Journals for Nature Cure, 38-9/1997. In combination with electro-neural-therapy and several methods of holistic therapy.

PART I

THE HISTORY OF THE PROBLEM

"Good," "Bad," and "Extreme-Bad"
Proteins—The Real Story

Chapter 1

THE PERFECT MATCH BETWEEN FOOD CHEMISTRY & BODY CHEMISTRY

The History of Good Protein and the Birth of "Bad" and "Extreme-Bad" Protein

It is no secret that we human beings have clear-cut rules about our biology and chemistry. And, of course, we all know that we are part of the zoological class Mammalia, which evolved from mammal-like reptiles roughly 200 million years ago.[9]

But what you may not know, and a crucial point to remember, is this: as mammals, our body chemistry—digestive system, metabolism, and enzymes—evolved from eating habits *over the course of millions of years.*

Even though we have gone through the most wondrous technical revolution the world has ever seen, we are still mammals. Nothing in our biology has changed in many, many millennia. We still give birth to live offspring the same as all of our kind. We still have the same digestion. The mouth is still the place where the splitting of starches and sugars begins. And we're still governed by the laws of body chemistry.

Yet, we know more about refrigerators, televisions, and computers than about our closest companion: our body.

Well, you may say, our brain—a biochemical drug factory composed of the most flexible matter in our body—has developed and changed and adapted dramatically. This is true, but the brain didn't change dramatically within a couple of decades. It took thousands and thousands of years to evolve. Generally, it takes a millennium for our bodies to undergo really dramatic changes.

But, we asked our BioChemical Machine to change within a couple of decades! Our body—which developed over the course of 200 million years—was supposed to adapt, within a relatively short space of time, to a radically changed world of supermarkets and fast food restaurants, where you just have to choose and your food is provided.

During the millions of years of mammalian development, there was no cooked meat or fish, no processed cheese, and no pasteurized and homogenized milk to bother anyone's body chemistry. There were only "good" proteins available, like those foods found in the "A" and Neutral columns of the A&B Chart.

---

*At this point, I would like you to keep the **A&B Chart** at hand. By glancing from time to time at this list, you will see that all food items are classified into three groups: either "A," "B," or Neutral (including "good" proteins.*

As you can see from the A&B Chart, Neutrals include not only salami, beef-salami, smoked and rolled ham, bacon, smoked sausages, beef jerky, smoked and marinated fish, beans, fava beans, lentils, all kinds of nuts, seeds, avocados, mushrooms, vegetables, salads, sprouts, olives, herbs, and blueberries—but also butter, oils, mayonnaise (no typo!), and a lot of dairy products, such as cream, heavy cream, sour cream, yogurt, whey, cottage cheese, mozzarella, Kefir, ewe's-milk cheese (such as Roquefort), goat's milk cheese (such as feta), Camembert, Brie, cream Gouda, and other cheeses *above* 60% fat.

If eaten properly—which means according to the natural laws of your body chemistry—Neutral food items, even the often-vilified dairy products, butter, and oils, do not cause health and weight problems. The even bigger bonus: you can eat *anything and at any time* from the Neutral group, *24 hours a day, 7 days a week.*

Good Proteins Gone Bad

But first things first. Let's delve into the history of the problem—the birth of the "bad" proteins. We'll begin with the most common belief about our more recent ancestors, *Homo erectus*, and the excuse for making cooked meat a major part of our diet.

They were supposed to be wild killer apes that ate primarily meat and that's why we are allegedly still doing the same. But the truth is, at no time were we near being a meat-devouring ape, as falsely maintained by anthropologists for 27 years.[10]

Homo erectus was not even primarily a hunter. Both men and women hunted only from time to time. Mostly, they were simple and peaceful gatherers of vegetables, fruits, seeds, and nuts, who mainly cracked bones left behind by predatory animals in order to eat the marrow.[10] Marrow is not only a good protein, but it also contains the number one energy supplier: fat.

For thousands of years, our ancestors ate foods like those found in the "A" and Neutral columns of the A&B Chart, which include "good" proteins, such as smoked or rolled ham, legumes, cured and dried meat, salami, and smoked fish. There were no historically new "bad" or "extreme-bad" proteins like those found in the "B"-column of the A&B Chart, such as low-fat or fat-free cheese, cooked meat, or cooked fish. Yet our ancestors' metabolism was satisfied. They got it all: carbohydrates, fats, and proteins. Why? Because most foods found in nature strike a consistent balance of carbohydrates, fats and proteins.

So, what makes a protein good or bad? When our ingenious ancestors invented the unique concept of cooking, it changed the nature of proteins. Every raw meat, fish, and milk and dairy product is Neutral by nature, creating no conflict within our body. The same is true for cured, dried, and smoked meat and fish.

It is the cooking process that changes (denatures) the chemistry of proteins, altering their sophisticated chain of amino acids. Exposure to high temperatures changes the chemistry of Neutral proteins and turns them into unhealthy acid-builders—the "extreme-bad" proteins that are so damaging to our health.

Our body chemistry, after only about a half century of eating this way, is still not adjusted to such hardship. Statistics like the 700% increase in U.S. diabetes cases over the last thirty years reflect this reality.[11]

Even our very recent ancestors, who domesticated animals and lived a very different life that included cooked meat—the "extreme-bad" proteins—didn't have the luxury of slaughtering one of their cows, goats, or sheep every day. Most people were poor and did not have several or even one animal. If they had livestock, it was reserved for festivals and special events. When an entire family or a village shared in the eating of one animal, each person got only a very small piece.

If there was enough left over, they dried, smoked and cured the meat. For thousands of years our ancestors have eaten very little meat, most of it preserved. These preserved foods, however, are Neutral proteins—the "good" proteins. This is why today's salami, rolled ham, pemmican (beef jerky), smoked bacon, and dried, smoked, or cured fish belong to the Neutral group. Rolled ham, for example, will be first cured and then stored in salt for three to four weeks. Afterwards, in order to ensure its durability, the ham will be dried and smoked, but not cooked. Other sausages, like salami, are made of uncooked muscle and fat but without adding water. They are preserved due to drying, smoking or curing—NOT cooking. The same is valid for any smoked, dried or cured food items.

At this point I would like to tell you about a real-life demonstration of the danger of "extreme-bad" protein consumption. In Tibet, it was once the custom not to immediately execute any person sentenced to death.

The Tibetans wanted a true punishment for those who undermined their society. To that end, the incarcerated felon was fed *nothing but cooked meat*.

We don't eat too much "extreme-bad" protein because we have been sentenced to death; we do it voluntarily. We eat much more protein than is required for tissue replacement. Why? During the 1950s and 1960s the rising meat industry hammered slogans like 'Eat meat. It's good for your energy' into people's minds. Soon, nobody doubted that a big man needs a big steak if he wants to be strong. But this is not the case.

As paradoxical as it may sound, it is entirely possible to develop a protein deficiency while eating too much cooked and fried meat-"extreme–bad" proteins. "Good" proteins are necessary for a healthy body. I'll say it again (because propaganda says otherwise): fat is the number one and carbohydrates the number two supplier of energy.

How should you know the laws of your body chemistry if you hear day in and day out all kinds of fairy tales about all kind of foods by companies that have turned you into a money-making machine? Yet the real problem is not that companies want to make money; the real problem is that you are, unknowingly, poisoning yourself slowly but surely. Paradoxically, companies will still make sufficient money once people begin to eat according to the laws of body chemistry.

Our body chemistry cannot change overnight. We need to find a solution to deal with the current reality; one that adjusts our modern eating habits to our old-fashioned digestive chemistry. And that's what the A&B Method is all about. Let's take human milk as an example of how Mother Nature meant us to eat.

Human breast milk is approximately 85% water. The remainder is 6.9% carbohydrates, 3.7% fat and 1.2% protein. We all know that there is no better food in this world than mother's milk for the first six months of life.

This ratio is indeed interesting, because, human milk is made up of the best energy suppliers: carbohydrates and fats. Only a small percentage of the milk is protein. In the final analysis, this ratio is exactly Mother Nature's concept for our eating habits.

What did the majority of our ancestors really do with their cows, goats or sheep, over the last 10,000 years? They drank the milk and produced (but did not pasteurize and homogenize) healthy dairy products like butter, cream, sour cream, buttermilk, all kind of curds (like the curdled cheese that we call today cottage cheese), and goat's or sheep's milk cheese (like feta)—which are all good protein sources.

Cow's milk would be Neutral in its original state. (That's why our ancestors ate compatibly by eating bread and drinking milk and milk products—thus "A" and Neutral). The pasteurizing and homogenizing process changes the chemistry of milk, so today, it falls into the "B"-column on the A&B Chart. But, despite pasteurizing and homogenizing, which means eating denatured protein, milk is still a moderate base-builder (a healthy, acid-nullifying food) *if* ingested with compatible foods from the "B"-column, especially apples and other "B"-fruits, and, of course, with Neutrals.

However, some dairy products are unhealthy acid-builders. Cheeses, which are below 50% fat like those found in the "B"-column are recent inventions, thus *new history.*

Our factories and methods of processing the new history foods became more sophisticated—and so did our cheese. It became a strong unhealthy acid-builder, a "bad" protein.

> **BioChemical Machine Fact**: *Modern food processing has had the same effects on carbohydrates like refined flour products and white-polished rice as well as fats like hardened margarine. I want to emphasize here that although new history foods are unhealthy acid-builders, their impact on health is not nearly as damaging as the "extreme-bad" proteins.*

As you will read throughout the book, the "bad" and "extreme-bad" proteins are emergency suppliers to our metabolism. By relying on either protein you will be satiated for the moment, especially at the beginning of dieting, but soon be very hungry, as it is a very poor fuel on which to support activity—expensive in every sense of the word. Yet it is no secret that almost every fad diet is based on too much of these "bad" and "extreme-bad" proteins. That's why fad diets leave you hungry.

You are not hungry because you decided to lose weight or because you are too weak to control your cravings (which leads to feelings of guilt). You are hungry because you and your metabolism *are* in fact starving. Hunger is a signal, a chemical reaction that your body didn't get what the metabolism needs to do its job: minerals, amino acids, fatty acids, enzymes, fats, carbohydrates and a small amount of "good" proteins from the Neutral group on the A&B Chart.

Yet, there are sufficient sources which will provide you with healthy protein, such as wheat bread, rye bread, brown rice, and, of course, base-builders such as fruits, vegetables, and salads. Ironically, the best and most high-grade protein is nowhere else but in the potato!

BioChemical Machine Fact: *The idea of "calories" stems from the time when the steam engine was born: put in coal and out comes energy. Unfortunately, today diet gurus would have us believe that it must be the same with food. One calorie is the unit of heat that is required to warm 1 gram of water from 14.5 to 15.5 degrees Celsius. That's all. It's just a measurement of heat. We are not steamboats; we are a more complicated BioChemical Machine, which adhere to the laws of our body's own chemistry.* **With the A&B Method, you do NOT need to count calories.**

And here we are. We are at the beginning of the journey that could change your life forever. The A&B Method will realign your body chemistry to the modern world. It is the perfect balance of food chemistry and body chemistry. By following the principles of the A&B Method, you will make a dramatic, fast, and long-term difference in your overall well-being. You will feel the difference within the first two weeks—its impact is that powerful. Your vitality will begin to return and heartburn, which is the direct result of excessive stomach acid in the lower esophagus, will start to disappear.

This immediate success is not as much astonishing as it is logical. As your unbalanced body chemistry begins to regulate itself, step-by-step your body will be able to get rid of the poisons you have accumulated and stored up, probably over the course of many years.

The next chapter will give you a clear picture why the perfect match of body chemistry and food chemistry is of such great significance; and how this match will ensure you never poison yourself again. With the A&B Method, your body will never return to a hyper-acidic state, but will instead maintain the vital *alkaline reserve*.

Therefore, let us discuss the cause of *Self-Poisoning: The Alkaline Deficit* and its impact on our health, energy, and body weight.

Chapter 2

THE ALKALINE DEFICIT:
A Road to Self-Poisoning

I am always astonished to hear people talking about guilt in connection with dieting and its relapse. How can anyone feel guilty about the desire to eat? Eating is one of the five basic human needs, along with drinking, breathing, sleeping and sex. How can anyone feel guilty about something that is stronger than our will? We are born with the desire to eat in order to live. No basic human need would ever create any problem for us as long as it didn't interfere with Mother Nature. But this is what we have done, and not only when it comes to food.

If anyone is "guilty," then it's our industrial revolution and prosperity itself. Do you want to blame yourself for the rise of the food industry and its seductive products? New food products require a new approach to matching food and body chemistry.

This new approach is crucial in dealing with all those alluring products found in supermarkets and restaurants. *We cannot turn back the clock.*

The food industry is part of our world. But we can learn to live in it in a way that leaves us healthy and energetic.

The Cell—Understanding the Problem

Our very existence is based on the cell*. If our cells are not healthy, we are not healthy. Our organs require healthy cells to function perfectly. The food we eat is responsible for the nourishment of our cells. Thus, we can decide the health of our cells and ourselves by eating according to the laws of your body chemistry.

But here's the catch: most people don't know about the perfect match of food and body chemistry. Therefore, they unknowingly disregard the laws of chemistry, build up acid after acid, and poison themselves. If you poison your body over many years by not eating correctly, you can be almost sure that you will develop serious illnesses later in life.

Fatigue is often the first indication that something is wrong with our cells and thus, our body chemistry. One-third of the U.S. population has difficulty staying awake after eating.[12] Often, the causes of fatigue are also harbingers of more serious problems. What's more, pathological fatigue is only one result of unknowingly poisoning yourself. Step by step, additional physical symptoms will arise, like coughing, headaches, swollen eyelids, dizziness, bloodshot eyes, and cloudy vision.

---

*The cell, in biology, is a discrete, membrane-bound portion of living matter. It is the smallest unit capable of an independent existence. All living organisms consist of one or more cells, with the exception of viruses.

But this is just the beginning. Starting around age thirty, human cell activity begins to slow and the regeneration process declines decade by decade. The immune system reduces its production of antibodies, leaving us more susceptible to sickness. Muscle mass is replaced by fat, unless we do something about it.

One day you will come to the point that it feels as if you body is falling apart. Probably you will pacify yourself with the common belief that pain after fifty is the fate of every human being on earth. But this is just not true. Once you know how to match food and body chemistry, you will have control over your health and energy, slowing down the aging process. You will not only have more fun during your early and middle years, but also really look forward to your "golden" years. As Dr. Hay says, "it is more a question of understanding foods and…at the same time respecting the laws of chemistry."[14]

Remember! If your cells are healthy, **you are healthy**. The food we eat and how we eat it makes all the difference. You will maximize the efficiency of your digestive system, which in turn will help maintain properly functioning metabolism. A strong metabolism will ensure that you will not be storing poisonous cells with their acidic end products. A healthy metabolism is also vital for your immune system; the decline of the metabolism creates a higher risk for infection and, ultimately, chronic diseases. "Disease never attacks healthy tissue; for the resistant body will not harbor infection, as it will not degenerate in structure and function," Dr. Quazi Al Tariq says.

A very, very sad statistic reflects this fact: "100,000 Americans will die [each year] because of wrong dieting."[3]

I began pondering the image of food. Food: what an ordinary thing. Even haute cuisine doesn't have the glamour of Cartier, Gucci, or Chanel. But without it you couldn't even think of Cartier, Gucci, and Chanel. Think about it. If we are arrogant in regard to our basic nature, we are poisoning ourselves. Did I say arrogant? Perhaps I should say ignorant, because we *would* respect our basic nature if we understood it. No one would voluntarily poison him or herself, creating a never-ending struggle with weight problems, chronic disease, pain, and even an early death.

This book is the instruction manual for the way your body—your BioChemical Machine—interacts with food. It's complicated if you don't know the laws of your body's chemistry; simple once you do. Therefore, let's talk about the underlying cause of so many problems relating to our health.

What Causes Self-Poisoning?

"Self-poisoning" goes by many names: over-acidification, toxification, intoxification, self-toxification, or toxemia. But all refer to the acidic end products of digestion and metabolism; your body's toxic waste.

There are TWO different ways your body creates this toxic waste: one that we cannot control and one that we can:

1. THE NORMAL PROCESS OF METABOLISM: Many of the billions of cells that make up our bodies die every day. They are constantly being replaced by new cells. The dead cells must be removed by one of our excretory organs: lungs, bowels, skin, liver, or kidneys as quickly as possible. A certain amount of these acidic end products are the result of the body's own decomposition and death. It is during this replacement process, that the acidic debris of dying cells accumulates in the body.

2. CREATING BODY CHEMISTRY IMBALANCE: If you burden your metabolism by eating *incompatible* foods that disregard the laws of your body chemistry, you are producing a surplus of poisonous cells that can't be excreted fast enough or incorporated into cell structures. Creating an accumulation of debilitating poisons in your system.

Many, if not most illnesses are related to the surplus of these metabolic-related toxic wastes that remain somewhere in your body instead of being eliminated through the skin, colon, liver and kidneys. The tissue residues determine illness or health. Disease rarely develops in normal tissues; those nourished with a proper blood supply and, thus, a higher degree of alkalinity.

The blood works according to very narrow parameters and sickness can quickly result if these parameters are not respected. "The blood, if not toxin-free, puts a tremendous strain upon the heart," says Dr. Al Tariq.[15] The same happens to be the case with the liver, lungs, pancreas, kidneys, thyroid gland, adrenal glands, and lymphatic system. Acid waste reaches the tissues almost always through blood and lymph toxicity.

> *BioChemical Machine Fact: Body chemistry is not negotiable. It must be respected in order to remain healthy, energetic, and free of pain. Your acid-alkaline reserve makes the difference.*

The Alkaline Reserve

I'm sure that many of you will ask the question "Why don't we immediately die from self-poisoning?" The answer is simple. We are a vigorous species, meant to survive. We are a biological masterpiece. Mother Nature allowed us to evolve from one single cell into hundreds of billions of cells. We limit ourselves by interfering with Mother Nature and her concept of our body chemistry.

In reality, it is a miracle that we are able to survive our modern eating habits while almost completely disregarding the laws of body chemistry. To make this miracle happen, Mother Nature equipped us with a safety net, a buffer system that makes the necessary adjustments.

"The alkaline* reserve acts as a buffer to maintain proper balance in the blood," explains Dr. Al Tariq.[16] This buffer is a mixture of chemical compounds chosen to maintain a steady pH** (the scale for measuring acidity or alkalinity).

There are several different buffer systems in our body and several organs have the capacity of a buffer system. The most common buffers consist of a weak organic acid and a mixture of salts of phosphoric acids. The addition of either an acid or a base causes a shift in the chemical equilibrium, thus keeping the pH constant.

Scientists began studying and quantifying the importance of the alkaline reserve in the laboratory to more fully understand the fluctuations of the content of CO^2 and HCO^3 in the blood. They documented the importance of this bicarbonate system. Further buffer systems in the blood are proteins and inorganic phosphates. Also lungs and kidneys provide buffer capacity. Blood, lungs and kidneys compensate for disturbances in the acid-alkaline balance of a healthy person. This is the way we are able to adapt to extreme situations, which we all do, day in and day out.

---

*ALKALINE: in our context, a substance having a pH above that of neutral water (7.0) when in solution. Signified as pH (potential of hydrogen), alkaline fluids, such as the blood (pH about 7.4), have the ability to neutralize acids (solutions below pH 7.0). Metabolic wastes are acids, and the alkaline reserve of the blood neutralizes them until they are excreted (Medical Dictionary).

**pH is the scale for measuring acidity or alkalinity. "From the standpoint of pure energy, pH is the measurement of electrical resistance between negative and positive ions in the body. The pH level is a measurement of the number of hydroxyl (OH-)ions which are negative and alkaline-forming, as opposed to the amount of hydrogen (H+) ions that are positive and acid-forming. Alkaline and acid-forming reactions are purely electro-chemical—i.e., pH measures how much the negative (alkaline-forming) ions and positive (acid-forming) ions push against one another," explains Dr. Al Tariq.[20]

But even this buffer system has its limit if we overburden our metabolism by disregarding the laws of our body's chemistry. The alkaline reserve is only a back-up system with limited capacity to keep you from constantly poisoning yourself.

> **BioChemical Machine Fact:** *Chronic alkaline deficit is a major reason for getting sick. Fatigue is the first sign that something is wrong with our body chemistry. But it also applies the other way around—when self-poisoning is gone then fatigue is gone.*

"The function of every organ and tissue depends on the height, breadth and depth of the alkaline reserve," explains Dr. Al Tariq.[17] "The lower the alkaline level, the lower the function. Conversely, the higher the alkaline reserve, the higher the level of activity our bodies can perform. The alkaline reserve is the body's bank account."[18]

I would add that it's more than a bank account, maybe better described as a savings account that the body can call upon anytime to release alkaline elements to neutralize harmful acids, but, there's a limit to how much can be saved. Since most people don't know this fact, they attempt to function with deficient alkaline reserves.

---

*Once, the scientific community believed that the body maintains its acid-alkaline balance through the buffer systems. It was believed that excessive carbonic acid would be exhaled through the lungs, and the kidneys would release the remaining acids directly, or in the form of easily soluble salts. Contemporary scientists proved the existence of the phenomenon of over-acidification.

The Alkaline Deficit

Therefore, let's talk about the corpus delicti, the cause for most of our problems: "The Alkaline Deficit," the result of Dr. Hay's revolutionary research about the acid-alkaline balance and alkaline reserve. Acid and alkaline are opposites that should be balanced. You should have neither too much alkaline in your blood nor too much acid. The alkaline reserve ensures that your body will be able to maintain this balance. It is responsible for binding these acids as they form and will decide how we live, even whether we live at all.

But what are acids? Are acids really as bad as described throughout this chapter? If we're talking about unhealthy acids, then the answer is yes. But we need to distinguish between healthy and unhealthy acids, because there are indeed acids your body needs, acids that are vital to good health:

STOMACH ACIDITY
Hydrochloric acid (HCl) is produced by the stomach to digest foods. It is an essential acid that is produced by our body as a natural process. Digestion produces stomach acids. All other acids are products of metabolism.

THE HEALTHY METABOLIC ACIDS
By nature, our body needs small portions of acid-building foods in order to fulfill certain tasks. For cxample, acid causes pain on the free nerve endings as an important warning signal. Pain indicates that something is wrong with our body.

Lactic acid and carbon dioxide originate in hardworking muscles and create the fatigue that warns us about excessive physical activity. The increase of carbon dioxide levels in the blood affects the way we breathe, so that more carbon dioxide will be exhaled through deeper breathing to restore the acid-alkaline balance.

THE UNHEALTHY METABOLIC ACIDS
The unhealthy acids, the cause of the alkaline deficit, are created by disregarding the A&B principles and eating too much of the "bad" and "extreme-bad" proteins. The right consumption amount is different for everyone. Healthy, active individuals should have no difficulties properly metabolizing these proteins. However, individuals suffering from serious health ailments must limit consumption of "bad" and "extreme bad" proteins—shaded gray and red on the A&B Chart LEVEL TWO—and denatured carbohydrates group III—shaded gray on the A&B Chart LEVEL TWO—to once a month and then only along with raw, fresh base-builders. You will read much more about this in subsequent chapters.

The Solution

But what is the solution to restoring your body's alkaline savings account? It's simple: smart dietary habits that build up and sustain an alkaline reserve. The only way alkaline and acid enter your body is by eating. Some foods will be metabolized into alkaline and others into acid.

If you don't eat according to the laws of your body chemistry, your BioChemical Machine will undergo undue hardship and eventually be "out of order."

I'm sure you will say, "You make it sound so easy, but seductive foods in every supermarket, deli, and fast food restaurant are just lurking around every corner, inviting me to eat and eat and eat. Who in the world can think of acid or alkaline when their mouth is watering?"

You are right; this is the dilemma of our modern world. But if you take a close look at the A&B Chart (LEVEL ONE for healthy people and LEVEL TWO for people with health problems and/or obesity and/or over 40) you'll see that you can eat almost anything you want—PROVIDED you match foods according to their chemical compatibility with your body.

LEVEL ONE
The first important step is to eat according to the A&B Method—the perfect match of food chemistry and body chemistry. Following these principles will make the quickest and largest difference.

LEVEL TWO
People with health and/or weight problems, or who are over 40, need to not only eat according to the A&B Method (LEVEL ONE) but also to follow the 80% base-builders/20% acid-builders ratio—avoiding, if not eliminating, the "bad" and "extreme-bad" proteins from their diet.

---

*Although the difference between acidosis and alkalosis seems to be very slight (as measured in terms of pH), this difference is vital to good health, energy, and weight control. Even a latent over-acidification of tissues with still normal alkaline reserve and normal acid-alkaline balance can pave the way for many illnesses.[19]

By following the A&B Method, you'll bring your weight under control, curtailing the effects of obesity, which brings with it a host of health nightmares. Obesity is linked to numerous disturbances of the metabolism, such as increased fat levels in the blood, kidney stones, varicose veins, disturbances of the blood circulation, and the risk of developing thrombosis and embolism. Excessive weight also burdens the spinal column and the hip and knee joints. It is well known that obesity is a risk factor for heart and circulatory diseases and for breast and colon cancer. Eventually, it leads to more frequent appearance of various forms of cancer.*

Knowledge is power. And knowledge of yourself means that you will have control over your health, weight, energy, and even over the speed of your aging process. Armed with the knowledge about the perfect match of food chemistry and body chemistry and its creation of the vital acid-alkaline balance, you will know what is right and what is wrong for your body. You don't need to study medicine or biochemistry in order to understand how your body works. The A&B Chart makes it easy to follow the principles of your body chemistry and to turn knowledge into practice. It's just a question of becoming conscious that we are a BioChemical Machine that needs to be treated right.

---

*In December 1998 the NBC show interviewed John J. Lynch of the American Cancer Society, who stated that "wrong diet was responsible for 40% of the cancer cases."[21] The American Cancer Society published in "Cancer Prevention & Early Detection," © 2000: "According to scientific research done over the past two decades, about one-third of all US cancer deaths can be attributed to the adult diet, including its effect on obesity."

As a side effect, many health and weight problems will simply disappear.

What did Dr. Hay say a hundred years ago? "When intoxification is gone then fatigue is gone...." When fatigue is gone, energy is back. And when energy is back, health is back. Nothing has changed since Dr. Hay's revolutionary discovery. This was the reality 200 million years ago, a hundred years ago, and it is valid for the six billion people who live today on this wonderful planet. It will be the reality as long as humans exist. No diet drink or high-protein diet can satisfy your metabolism because our organs and glands function properly in exact proportion to the amount of alkaline and acid levels in the system. Yet we are still running after the mirage that any fad diet of miracle pill could satisfy such a sophisticated machine like ours.

In Chapter 3, you'll learn more about how your sophisticated *BioChemical Machine* operates.

PART II

THE
A&B PRINCIPLES

Balancing The BioChemical Machine

Chapter 3

THE BIOCHEMICAL MACHINE
Understanding the Role of Digestion

Self-poisoning does not occur overnight. It takes years, if not decades of making bad choices to build up toxins—poison—in our BioChemical Machine. Unfortunately, we don't immediately feel the extent of the damage because our species is equipped to survive. On one hand, this is great; on the other, that's exactly where the danger lies. If we immediately became ill when we ate incorrectly, we would learn very quickly to always eat right.

Our body has a tremendous power to correct itself. This correction begins with the food we eat. At the heart of your body's delicate biochemical balance is food and the way it is digested. As the distribution center of your well-being, digestion nourishes cells, enzymes, metabolism, tissues, blood, the lymphatic system, and all organs.

Without digestion, there is no energy. And without energy, there is no life. In short, it is the center of your very existence.

Gaining control over your digestion can change your life forever. It empowers your metabolism to do a proper and efficient job, enabling it to cleanse your body of poisoned cells and acidic end products. So understanding the digestive process is an important starting point.

Let's begin by examining the different ways your body digests different foods—and why foods are categorized the way they are on the A&B Chart.

1. NEUTRAL PROTEIN DIGESTION
The "Good" Proteins

Neutral proteins—the foods found in the middle column of the A&B Chart like uncooked meats, fish (smoked, cured, etc.) and dairy products which have not been homogenized or pasteurized, as well as uncooked or cooked egg yolks—are "old history," so much a part of our biological nature through the millennia that your body has no trouble digesting them. They can be eaten at any time with foods from the "A" **or** "B"-column or any other item in the Neutral group on the A&B Chart.

2. "B"-PROTEIN DIGESTION
The "Bad" and "Extreme-Bad" Proteins

Acid-building proteins like those found in the "B"-column of the A&B Chart are easy to digest PROVIDED you don't ask your body to do so with other foods from either the "A" and "B"-columns at the same time.

Digestion of the new history foods—"B"-proteins like cooked meats, eggs, cheeses below 50% fat, and pasteurized and homogenized milk, causes acid to build up in your body–which as you now know, deducts from the important alkaline reserve. But as long as you don't eat incompatible foods as defined by the A&B Chart, your body can cope.

To make the digestion of "B"-proteins—the historically new "bad" and "extreme-bad" proteins—possible, the stomach's gastric juice needs to be very acidic. "B"-protein digestion begins in the stomach with an enzyme called pepsin, in the presence of hydrochloric acid. Without the action of pepsin, those acid-building "B"-proteins couldn't go through the first step of digestion.

BioChemical Machine Fact: The enzyme pepsin will act only in an acidic environment.

It's during this first step that "B"-proteins are reduced to amino acids and peptides. However, starches (complex carbohydrates), sugars, and fats are not digested by these gastric juices. The second step in this digestion process takes place in the small intestine. It's there that the "B"-protein digestive process is completed by pancreatic juice, intestinal juice, and bile. The pancreatic juice contains the enzymes trypsin, amylase and lipase that are vital to completing this process.

3. CARBOHYDRATE DIGESTION

Unlike the acid-building "B"-proteins, carbohydrates must have alkaline conditions to be digested.

Chewing is the very important first and most underrated step in digesting carbohydrates. In addition to the fact that digestive juices can react more easily to finer particles of food, saliva is essential to breaking down carbohydrates. Why? Saliva contains an enzyme called amylase; its role is to split the complex carbohydrate and sugars into smaller units or simple sugars.

> **BioChemical Machine Fact:** *The enzyme, amylase, will act only in a positive alkaline environment.*

After the food is swallowed, it passes through the esophagus into the stomach where it mixes with amylase and is reduced into simple sugars, ready for intestinal digestion. If the environment isn't at least slightly alkaline, digestion will be hindered and starches will reach the small intestine almost undigested.

Digestion continues in the small intestine where additional amylase generated from the pancreas and secreted from the walls of the small intestine, decompose the remaining starches into simple sugars.

Again, if the environment of the small intestine isn't lightly alkaline, allowing the amylase to do its work, then digestion will be hindered. One consequence is a buildup of gases, which cause the infamous feeling of fullness, fatigue, and pain.

> **BioChemical Machine Fact:** *The enzymes pepsin (required for "B"-protein digestion) and amylase (required for carbohydrate digestion) counteract each other's action when put together.*

By eating different types of foods that require two different types of digestion ("A" and "B" columns at the same time), we make it difficult for our bodies to efficiently digest food. We are also creating a chaotic situation for the mixing chamber, the stomach. The stomach cannot be both acidic and alkaline at the same time. As stated before, the enzyme amylase can function only if sufficient alkaline is available. Without the stimulation of this alkaline medium there is no action of the enzyme amylase on carbohydrates. Even the slightest acid reaction can slow down the splitting process of carbohydrates and can go so far as to arrest the process of starchy reduction.

When we eat chemically incompatible foods together, digestion is not only made more difficult but is considerably delayed. We may even make it impossible to digest the foods completely. As stated before, when we put conflicting enzymes together during the digestive process they are unable to function properly.

4. FAT DIGESTION

Advertisers have invested huge sums of money and time into making you believe the slogan "fat makes fat." This fallacy has become big business in regard to your health. The truth is, because of their chemical makeup, all fats and oils fall under the Neutral category on the A&B Chart.

Unlike "B"-proteins and carbohydrates, fats and oils don't require special treatment to prepare them for digestion in the small intestine.

Although the stomach and small intestine secrete fat-decomposing enzymes, those enzymes' significance is small.

The pancreas does most of the work by secreting the enzyme pancreas-lipase into the duodenum, where, with the help of liver-produced bile, the fats are broken down and emulsified into a soapy form and easily absorbed into the bloodstream. To further support the work of your metabolism to break down fats, eat foods that contain healthy supplies of Pantothenic acid. The vitamins contained in Pantothenic acid play a central role in demolishing fat. Pantothenic acid is available in vegetables, especially cauliflower (which detoxifies cells and creates new skin) and mushrooms, but it is also found in whole wheat bread, nuts and yeast.

Now that you have a better understanding of how different foods are digested differently, let's examine how we can utilize this knowledge to properly balance your BioChemical Machine.

Chapter 4

HEALTHY LIVING
WITHOUT DIETS

Using the A&B Chart

Dispense with the magic pills promising a quick fix, the fad diets that don't work, the deprivation that leaves you hungry and unhappy. The A&B Method is about what you should eat—not what you shouldn't—based on your body chemistry.

The A&B Method is all about learning how to contend with and even reverse the health-damaging effects caused by the new history, "bad" and "extreme-bad" proteins. As discussed earlier, this group of proteins is responsible for most—if not all—health and weight problems because they create excessive acidity, thereby reducing the effectiveness of digestive enzymes and ultimately undermining your alkaline reserve. If you choose foods based on their compatibility, then your BioChemical Machine will be kept in perfect balance and you will enjoy all the benefits of good health.

The A&B Chart was developed to give you all the information you need to make the right choices based on your physical condition. Everyone is different. How you use the A&B Chart will depend on different factors, like age, weight, and current health.

If you are under forty, at your ideal weight, and in good health, you can eat virtually anything you want, PROVIDED you match foods according to their chemical compatibility: "A"-column with Neutral, "B"-column with Neutral, **but never foods from the "A" and "B"-column together at the same meal.**

THIS IS LEVEL ONE OF THE A&B METHOD.

Base-Builder or Acid Builder?
It's As Easy as Yellow, White, Gray and Red

In LEVEL TWO of the A&B Method, the foods under each column on the A&B Chart are shaded yellow, white, gray or red. This was done to help you distinguish between foods that are base-builders and those that are acid-builders. If you have health and/or weight problems or if you are over 40, then you need to pay special attention to the color coordination on the LEVEL TWO A&B Chart. In addition to following the principles behind the "A," "B," and Neutral columns, you will also want to choose foods that create a diet balanced of 80% base-builders to 20% acid-builders.

A good rule of thumb to remember is:

Eat plenty from the YELLOW.
Eat moderately from the WHITE.
Avoid the GRAY and RED.

YELLOW: *Very Healthy Base-Builders*

The foods you find shaded yellow on the A&B Chart are the strong and moderate base-builders that should make up the backbone of your diet. The strong base-builders are vital for your alkaline reserves and should be the major component of each day's menu, while moderate base-builders are still strong enough to increase alkalinity. Like strong base-builders, the moderates may be part of each day's base-building foods.

WHITE: *Healthy Acid-Builders*

Moderate acid-builders are the acid-builders that your body needs, ideally eaten together with base-builders. Remember, not all acids are bad. Your body needs small portions of certain acid-building foods in order to fulfill important tasks.

GRAY & RED: *Unhealthy Acid-Builders*

The "new history" foods are the unhealthy acid-builders. The way in which they are processed and prepared have made them bad, bad, bad and we could live without them—if they didn't taste so good! Some of these acid-builders are more damaging than others. They are the cooked meats shaded red under the "B"-

column. If you are in good health, your body can absorb the costs of eating the occasional hamburger but, if you are overweight, suffering from disease, or over 40, the cost to your body chemistry really isn't worth it. So, try not to eat too much of the unhealthy acid-builders especially the "extreme bad" proteins from the "B"-column which are the worst of the worst. If you do choose to eat from the gray or red group, religiously follow the A&B principles and eat them with strong base-builders such as fruits, vegetables, and salads.

Learning To Live With ALL Foods

As you can see, carbohydrates, proteins, and fats are found in all columns of both the LEVEL ONE and LEVEL TWO programs, as well as in each of the yellow, white, gray, and red color schemes. Gurus that demand you eliminate fat or carbohydrates from your diet to lose weight are simply wrong. All the food groups—carbs, fats, and even proteins—are valuable parts of a balanced diet, provided you abide by the A&B principles, which distinguish between the good and the bad in each.

For example, carbohydrates shaded yellow on the A&B chart, such as potatoes, kale, millet, honey, sprouted grains, bananas, grapes, fresh figs, fresh dates, dried apples, dried plums, dried figs, dried dates, and raisins, are excellent base-builders. They are very healthy and may be eaten without limit.

> **BioChemical Machine Fact**: *Conventional wisdom has maintained that eating potatoes is a bad idea if you're trying to lose weight. Not so! Rich in vitamin and mineral content and packed with high-grade protein that provides essential amino acids, the potato is a strong base-builder and may be—even should be—eaten as often as possible. As long as you abide by the A&B principles, you may eat potatoes to your heart's content.*

However, not all carbohydrates are base-builders. Take for example natural, but *processed* carbs like whole wheat bread. Our bread is refined and cooked at temperatures above 300 degrees Fahrenheit changing it from a strong base-builder into a moderate acid-builder (at the boundary of being a moderate base-builder).[22] However, meat cooked at this temperature would turn it into an "extreme-bad" protein. These modern preparations cause the oxidation of wheat bread, which is why it releases carbonic acid into your system. Although it is relatively little acid in comparison to the following group, it should be eaten in the right proportion *with fresh base-builders.*

The same oxidation is true for grains such as natural rice, rye, oats and corn, all of which are rich in vitamins and minerals. If compatibly eaten, they too are most definitely a healthy choice. As such, you'll find them— along with whole wheat bread—included in the white group on the LEVEL TWO A&B Chart.

Not All Carbohydrates are Created Equal

But not all carbohydrates are good for you. Unnatural or denatured carbs—bleached and radically altered grains like refined white flour and processed sugar—are strong acid-builders. When these concentrated carbohydrates are metabolized, large amounts of carbonic acid are released into the body (although their debris is not as toxic as the "bad" and "extreme bad" proteins).

They, of course, are the carbohydrates shaded gray on the LEVEL TWO A&B Chart.

Young and healthy people may eat moderately from this group as long as they follow the principles behind the "A," "B," and Neutral columns. But if you are over 40, obese, or struggling with health problems, eating foods from the gray group should be a rare occurrence.

BioChemical Machine Fact: You need five to ten times the quantity of white bread (as compared with whole wheat bread) just to feel satiated. White bread has no substantial food value. In the final analysis, it is even more expensive than whole wheat bread.

As we have explored throughout the book, when we eat natural foods in their natural forms we are not troubled with acid formation. Nature balances these foods very nicely for our digestive abilities and keeps our body chemistry in harmony.

It is when we diverge from what nature intended that we upset the balance of our BioChemical Machine and poison ourselves, gradually and unknowingly.

Yet we don't need to starve our body of the right foods, causing health and weight problems, because we have the power to choose correctly. By following the A&B Methods, guided by LEVEL ONE or LEVEL TWO of the A&B Chart, you're on your way to perfect body chemistry and good health.

Chapter 5

THE BIG SEVEN ESSENTIALS
Balancing Body Chemistry

Now that you have an understanding of how your body chemistry reacts to different foods, let's get down to ways you can use this information for your benefit. In this chapter, I've distilled the essence of the A&B Method into seven essential steps. By incorporating these seven essentials into your day-to-day life, you'll *immediately* feel better and have more energy. You'll gain control of your appetite. Heartburn will disappear. In the long term, serious health and weight problems will improve and you'll even slow the aging process.

Is it really this simple? It can be, because your body chemistry is comprehensible, but not negotiable.

Neutrals can be eaten at any time, 24 hours a day, 7 days a week. But during the same meal, **don't eat foods from the "B"-group with foods from the "A"-group** because your BioChemical Machinery is just not made for it! This is the fundamental principle of the A&B Method and the key to a healthy and energetic life.

Eliminating the practice of eating foods from both the A&B columns during the same meals will result in an immediate boost to your alkaline reserve. In many cases, people have experienced the benefits within the first two weeks! This simple adjustment of your eating habits increases the effectiveness of your metabolism and jump-starts the process of cleansing your body of poisonous dead cells.

Essential #2
Replace "Bad" Protein
With healthy "Good" Protein

All proteins are not created equal. As discussed, consuming excess amounts of the acid-building "bad" and "extreme-bad" "B"-proteins is the likely cause of many of today's health problems. When cooked, foods from the "B"-column leave behind *the greatest amount* of the most irritating debris in your body; a wide array of very acidic and very irritating salts, chief of which is uric acid. Urea and uric acid remain in the body up to the time of excretion through the kidneys.

These two acids shift the acid-base balance toward acid (poison). At this stage, your body simply requires time to excrete the acid surplus.

However, as you know from Chapter 3, if your body is contending with digesting foods from both the "A" and "B"-columns at the same time, then you put an unnecessary burden on the buffer system-your alkaline reserve. As such, the body cannot excrete the acid surplus, because the blood is unable to buffer the masses of accrued acids coming in waves. This build-up of acids causes self-poisoning and leads to the host of health problems we've discussed.

The A&B Chart will help you distinguish between "good" and "bad" and "extreme-bad" proteins:

GOOD PROTEINS: The Neutral healthy proteins—found in the middle column of the A&B Chart and highlighted in white.

"BAD" & "EXTREME-BAD" PROTEINS: The unhealthy proteins—found in the "B"-column of the A&B Chart and highlighted in gray and red.

Don't be confused that whole milk is included in the "B"-column, despite the fact that milk is a moderate base-builder (boosting the alkaline reserve), thus healthy. Originally, whole milk was indeed a strong base-builder and belonged to the Neutrals. Modern pasteurizing and homogenizing changed the chemistry of milk. So, we should no longer drink milk along with foods from the "A"-column of the A&B Chart, such as bread, or potatoes. However, whole milk is still one of the best foods to detoxify the body in the morning.

Milk remains, despite pasteurizing, a moderate base-builder and a good protein source. What's more, increasing numbers of supermarkets are selling whole milk that is free of hormones and unnecessary chemicals.

What are the results of eating "bad" and "extreme-bad" proteins? As an example, let's take the diseases osteoporosis and arthritis. Remember that strong acid-building food, like cooked meat, shifts the pH balance in the body toward acid. If the body cannot buffer the acid in its blood, it will take vital minerals from the bones. The body is forced to mobilize calcium, magnesium and potassium from its reserves to balance the bases and acids in the blood and cells. Over time, over-acidification of the blood can lead to the degeneration of the bones.

Even though the body has vital alkaline reserves that neutralize acids, the fewer acids we create, the fewer bases we withdraw from our body's alkaline reserves. Eating too much "bad" and "extreme-bad" protein drains our alkaline reserves.

Time (November 24, 1997, No. 22, page 83) reported in the Health sector that "a landmark study" has shown that vegetarians had higher blood levels of lipoprotein "a." Furthermore, "a new analysis by a joint US-Italian team shows . . . that the fish eaters have an average 40% lower level of this particular lipoprotein."

| Essential #3 |
| Eat More of the Right Food: |
| Base-Builders and Healthy Carbohydrates |

Your food choices should be rich with the right kinds of food—plenty of the base-builders that you'll find highlighted in white and yellow in all three columns of the A&B Chart. "Good" proteins can be eaten 24/7. The only exception to this would be for those following LEVEL TWO where 80% of the food must be **FRESH** base-builders. Healthy "good" proteins are highlighted in white on the Neutral column of the A&B Chart.

Along with fats, carbohydrates are main suppliers of energy and rich in necessary fiber. We need to eat carbohydrates. However, in order to do what's best for our bodies, it's important to distinguish between three groups of carbohydrates: Group I, II, and III.

GROUP I—Yellow on the A&B Chart

These are the base-building carbohydrates. They may be eaten in unlimited amounts as long as you abide by the A&B principles.

GROUP II—White on the A&B Chart

These natural, but processed carbohydrates may be eaten daily, but, to play it safe, they should be eaten with base-builders, such as vegetables, salads, and compatible "A"-fruits.

These are the unhealthy carbohydrates. Yet they are NEVER as unhealthy as "bad" and "extreme-bad" proteins, whose toxic debris is VERY harmful. Whatever fairytale you have been told, chocolate, eaten compatibly, is never as unhealthy as a sausage on a bun or hamburger on a roll.

Essential #4
When It Comes to Carbohydrates
Chew, Chew, Chew

As you know, saliva is needed for the first step in carbohydrate digestion because it contains amylase, whose primary duty is to split the starches (complex carbohydrates) and sugars into smaller units or simple sugars. The more you chew, the easier it is for your body to properly digest carbohydrates.

Chewing is vital to properly digesting carbohydrates; ideally, 25 to 40 times per bite, according to the latest research.

Essential #5
Enhance Liver Function
with the Right Eating Schedule

The liver is responsible for regulating so many bodily functions that it is often referred to as "the custodian of the interior milieu." One of the liver's most important jobs is to remove damaged cells and toxins from the blood.

Yes, it is your liver that works hard to get rid of the poison created by your daily metabolism. And like you, it doesn't want to be bothered while working hard. So, support your liver! How? The liver has a natural rhythm, choosing the right time of day to eat certain foods will enhance its efficiency and function. Scientists refer to this as the biological liver rhythm*. In order to maximize on this natural rhythm, follow the A&B Method and eat:

- Base-builders in the morning, such as milk (or yogurt) and apples or other "B"-fruits, or only fruit, if you don't like milk or yogurt

- Healthy good proteins from the Neutral or "B"-group at midday

- Carbohydrates from the "A"-group along with Neutral foods in the afternoon and evening

---

Essential #6:
Breathing Correctly Is As
Important As Eating and Drinking

Correct breathing has far more impact on our health than generally assumed. Deep breathing exercises massage the abdominal region, which in turn, improves both blood circulation and the lymphatic system. This aids your metabolism and thereby the metabolism of fat. If you workout on a regular basis you already benefit from deep breathing.

---

*The biological liver rhythm is based on extensive research conducted by Swedish researcher Eric Abraham Forsgren.[23]

For the inactive crowd, set aside a few moments each day to take 100 deep, deep breaths. Lie down and take in slow deep breaths, first expanding your stomach and then filling your lungs. Aside from improving your blood and lymphatic system, you will feel greatly refreshed. A good investment of 5-10 minutes!

Essential #7:
Focus On Chemistry; Not Counting Calories

The A&B Method is NOT A DIET, so throw counting calories out the window. Diets are a temporary measure—no one stays on a diet forever, right?

The A&B Method is about knowledge. Knowing how your body works and how the fuel you put into your BioChemical Machine makes it run will serve you for the rest of your life. As long as you eat foods that are chemically compatible with your body chemistry, your body will respond by naturally returning to its ideal state: the perfect weight, full of energy, and pain free.

The BIG SEVEN ESSENTIALS

1• You Can Eat Neutrals 24 hours a day, 7 days a week. Eat from Group "A"—Eat from Group "B" But **AVOID** Eating Both at the Same Meal.

2• Replace "Bad" Protein with "Good" Protein

3• Eat More of the Right Foods: Base-Builders and Healthy Carbohydrates

4• When It Comes to Carbohydrates Chew, Chew, Chew

5• Enhance Liver Function with the Right Eating Schedule

6• Breathing Correctly Is As Important As Eating and Drinking

7• Focus On Chemistry; Not Counting Calories

PART III

DANGEROUS MISCONCEPTIONS

Chapter 6

Big FAT Myths:
The Important Role of Fat

As stated earlier, the myth that "fat makes fat" is at best untrue, at worst potentially dangerous. It also happens to be one of the diet industry's best moneymaking ideas.

In fact, fat is the body's number one energy reserve supplier, making it very important to our overall health. Fats, oils, fat-containing foods, and yes, even saturated fats play an important role in nourishing our BioChemical Machine. It stores energy, insulates body tissues, and transports fat-soluble vitamins to the blood, as well as plays a key role in cell structure and hormone production. Fat helps develop healthy bones and protects our organs from harm.

> **BioChemical Machine Fact:** *Fats can reduce high cholesterol. The body needs fat to function properly.*

Yet "fat makes fat" has been hammered into our minds, until we finally accepted the idea of our bodies being a sort of bacon-rind, a combination of lean meat with excess fat that must be eliminated by burning it off. Gurus will have you believe that a simple exercise session or two each and every day will burn away the fat and calories and solve all your health and weight problems.

It sounds like a logical association: fry a piece of bacon and it becomes liquid fat—fat that can be poured off. That's how we came to imagine our bodies to work. Exercise and sweat, and the fat will burn and burn and burn, so that it somehow will disappear, right? But in and of itself, this is not the case.

As we have seen, according to their chemistry, fats and oils belong to the Neutral group. They do not require special treatment to prepare them for digestion in the small intestine.[24]

If you follow the A&B principles, healthy fat will not make you fat. The truth is that a total of 60 to 80 grams (3–4 ounces) of healthy fats and oils is the correct daily amount for a healthy, moderately active person. Try to figure out how much you can eat over the course of a day to reach a total of 3 to 4 ounces of fat. You will be surprised.*

---

*If you have already developed a disease, you should discuss the quantity of fats and oils with your doctor.

However, there is a vast difference between healthy and unhealthy fats. The trick is knowing the difference.

UNHEALTHY FATS:
Industrialized fats, especially trans fat (trans fatty acid), whether they are saturated or unsaturated, are unhealthy fats. Trans fat is a human made substance (generally used by restaurants to fry chicken, French fries, etc. because it's cheap). Trans fatty acids disrupt cellular functioning.

HEALTHY FATS:
Healthy fats are natural, cold-pressed oils or virgin oils (no heat, no chemicals). Since these oils aren't subjected to the refining process, they are rich in vitamins and essential acids.

All natural, unsaturated oils are rich in the essential fatty acids vital to your body's ability to carry out important functions. Of all vegetable oils, linseed (flaxseed) and olive oil are the healthiest.

BioChemical Machine Fact: Research suggests that olive oil is especially beneficial when it comes to the heart. Olive oil protects against heart disease by acting as an anticoagulant that thins the blood and cuts the chance of blood clots or stroke-threatening blockages from forming.[25] It also lowers blood pressure. Research at the University of Texas Health Science Center reported that olive oil lowered dangerous LDL* cholesterol by 21 percent in middle-aged men. At the same time, it preserved good HDL** cholesterol levels.[25]

---

*LDL=Low Density Lipoprotein
**HDL=High Density Lipoprotein

Fat Free or Low-Fat Products

Whatever the reason, a misguided attitude about fat has led most to people believe that "fat-free" or "low-fat" products are the solution to their health and weight problems.

But buying into the fat-free, low-fat myth prevents you from eating healthy fats—an enormous problem. According to a study by the American Heart Association, "…very low fat diets can increase a person's bad cholesterol and rob them of essential nutrients, like iron and calcium." Dr. Linda van Horn, also of the American Heart Association concluded, "low fat diets can be dangerous, and potentially cause harm."[26]

The AHA is not alone in its assessment. Dr. Nancy Ernst of the National Institutes of Health states: "When you leave the fat at the shelf you left the vitamins and minerals also."[26] What's more, the food industry puts an *enormous* amount of sugar in these low-fat products to make them simulate natural fats and taste better (according to a 1999 CBS News report, "thirteen tablespoons of sugar, corn syrup are added to low-fat yogurt.")

Meddling with food chemistry doesn't stop there. Processing neutral cream cheeses, sour cream, yogurt, and curd, such as cottage cheese, into low-fat/nonfat/fat-free products turns them into unhealthy acid-builders—the "bad" protein (shaded gray on the A&B Chart in the "B"-column).

If you follow the A&B principles, you may eat butter and all Neutral milk products like cream, sour cream, cheese above 60% fat, cottage cheese, and, of course, the very healthy natural olive oil, sunflower oil, soy oil, linseed (flaxseed) oil, and sesame oil. These are the fats and oils that your metabolism needs.

Margarine or Butter

Many people choose margarine over butter, acting on the erroneous assumption that it is the healthy choice. I've often heard, "I prefer margarine because it contains unsaturated fat—because it is a vegetable product."

What they often forget is that in contrast to butter, margarine is an artificial product. "Although a vegetable product, and neutral, the use of commercial margarine is not recommended," explains the expert, Professor Leitzmann.[27] "The heating process breaks hydrogen bonds creating a product that causes rancidity and hardening in the tissues. Soy margarine is a slightly improved substance, but it is still not recommended in any large quantity." In addition, trans fatty acids are formed when vegetable oils are processed into margarine.[28] No question about it, butter is a base-builder, thus recommended over margarine.

Saturated Fat

Another myth I'm sure you've heard is about the evils of saturated fat. Yet if you carefully examine the foods that contain saturated fatty acids—meat and poultry, whole or reduced-fat milk, butter and some vegetable oils like coconut, palm kernel oil, and palm oil[28]—you'll see that something is drastically wrong with the saturated fat hysteria. Butter, coconuts, and whole milk are strong base-builders, as healthy as it gets! Animal fat is not the villain. Rather, it is the COOKED meat and the LACK of healthy fat in reduced-fat milks and cheeses that cause the harm, not butter and whole milk which are healthy base-builders.

BioChemical Machine Fact: The A&B Method is about what you should eat; NOT what you shouldn't eat.

Common misconceptions about nuts provide another example of how wrong ideas become generally accepted. Nuts are known to be very high in fat content, no question about it, yet they play a role in demolishing fat.

Another example is the often-vilified pizza. Even when its dough is made from refined white flour*, if its topping consists of ingredients from the Neutral column—like mushrooms, olives, onions, peppers, and mozzarella (or other cheese above 60% fat)—pizza remains a compatible meal. Only when you add tomato sauce (made from cooked tomatoes), cooked sausages, and pasta sauces with meat from the "B"-column do you violate the laws of your body chemistry.

The truth about fat is not as simple as the myth that has been created around it. I often read baffling advice about fat from diet gurus. For example, one guru asserts that "fat retards the digestion of protein," so it should be eaten with carbohydrates. Another diet guru demands exactly the opposite: only proteins should be combined with fat.

---

*People with health problems—LEVEL TWO—are strongly advised to eat a pizza made of whole wheat dough

Why would fat retard digestion? Fats and oils do not require any treatment to prepare them for digestion by the small intestine.[29]

Of course, you can bake your Thanksgiving turkey with butter, and, of course, you can pour butter with herbs over your fish filet. You can even indulge in bacon and eggs (yolks only) if you wish. And, of course, you can eat whole wheat bread with mayonnaise, tomatoes, and onions or baked potatoes with butter, dill, salt and pepper. And there is nothing wrong with eating natural rice with fried onions; spaghetti with butter, mushrooms, cream and peas; or banana flambé. The issue is to maintain the acid-alkaline balance by carefully following the A&B Chart.

Fat doesn't make you fat; rather, the lack of fat deprives you of important vitamins and minerals and can contribute to cell degeneration and illness. Your metabolism will function perfectly if you choose the right foods as outlined by the A&B Method. If you have reached the age when cells slow down, and/or if you have developed a chronic disease, then abide by the LEVEL TWO chart which emphasizes 80% base-builders and 20% acid-builders and avoid the "bad" and "extreme-bad" proteins.

Otherwise, you can dispense with the myths you've heard about fat. Understanding the match between food chemistry and body chemistry ensures that you know more than the diet gurus. That's how you will stay slim, energetic, healthy, and happy.

Chapter 7

THE TRUTH ABOUT CHOLESTEROL

And What You Don't Know About Homocysteine

It seems like every time we hear about cholesterol and saturated fat, it's linked to some ad promoting the latest and greatest "magic pill." In an interview on ABC's *20/20*, Dr. Thomas James, then president of the American Heart Association stated that a single anti-cholesterol drug released that year, from one of the major pharmaceutical manufacturers, generated "a *three billion dollar positive cash flow.*"[30]

Cholesterol has become big business. But is it true that it's as big a nutritional devil as we've been led to believe? And is it true that saturated fat is responsible for dangerously high cholesterol in the blood? Not entirely.

As is true with fat, there are a lot of misconceptions about cholesterol. The fact is, cholesterol is vital for the immune system and nearly all body cells. It is an integral part of all cell membranes and is a required component for building cell walls. It is the starting point for the production of steroid hormones, including the sex hormones. And you may be surprised to learn that cholesterol—once it is broken down by the liver into bile salts—helps your body decompose fat.[31] Two-thirds of your body's cholesterol is produced in your own liver.* The rest comes from the foods we eat.

But not all cholesterol is the same. There are two different kinds that function in your body.

HDL: The Good Cholesterol

Cholesterol is an essential component of lipoproteins, which transport fats and fatty acids in the bloodstream to tissues throughout the body. High-density lipoprotein (HDL) cholesterol acts as a scavenger, transporting fat and cholesterol from the tissues to the liver. Most of the cholesterol in the blood is in the form of high-density lipoproteins and can protect against arterial disease. HDL picks up cholesterol in the arteries and takes it back to the liver for excretion or reprocessing. HDL is often referred to as "good cholesterol."

---

*The liver has many regulatory and storage functions. It receives the products of digestion, converts glucose to glycogen (as long-chain carbohydrates used for storage), and breaks down fats. It removes excess amino acids from the blood, converting them to urea, which is excreted by the kidneys. The liver also synthesizes vitamins, produces bile and blood-clotting factors, and removes damaged red cells and toxins, such as alcohol, from the blood.

LDL: What You Don't Know About Bad Cholesterol.

You're probably already familiar with low-density lipoprotein (LDL), the so-called "bad cholesterol." According to conventional wisdom, saturated fat in the diet increases the LDL, which, in turn increases the risk of heart disease." While it is true that LDL, in excess, can become deposited on the surface of the arteries, which in turn can lead to arteriosclerosis, it is not true that this can be avoided simply by omitting saturated fat from your diet. If this were the case, than strict vegetarians would never have high cholesterol or suffer from heart disease.

Even if unsaturated fat-acids lower the cholesterol in the blood, it does not mean that omitting saturated fats makes everything all right. The truth is that your body can easily process saturated fat, as it can your own production of cholesterol, as long as your metabolism is functioning as it should.

All body functions are interrelated like stones in a mosaic. Take away one stone and the picture becomes less than perfect. Eliminating saturated fat from your diet is not the answer to high cholesterol. In fact doing so may affect your body chemistry adversely in other ways.

- Recent studies at the University of California at Los Angeles (UCLA) were conducted in which cholesterol levels in the blood were reduced by retaining it in the intestine (and interrupting its absorption into the bloodstream). Yet doing so resulted in only 1.8% fewer heart attacks—while the incidence of cancer increased by 5%.

Homocysteine: Another Stone in the Mosaic

In the big picture of your health, it's not only LDL cholesterol that can damage arteries and lead to heart attacks and stroke. An amino acid called homocysteine can play a part as well. High homocysteine levels in the blood can cause cholesterol to change to something called oxidized low-density lipoprotein, which is more damaging to the arteries than LDL. In addition, high homocysteine levels can make blood clot more easily than it should, increasing the risk of blood vessel blockages. A blockage can cause strokes or interrupt blood flow. Up to 20% of people with heart disease have high homocysteine levels.

According to Dr. Kilian Robinson of the Cleveland Clinic, "You can have normal cholesterol and normal blood pressure, but high homocysteine is often the only detectable reason why you might experience a vascular episode, heart attack or stroke."[30] He added, "high homocysteine may be just as important and widespread as a cardiac factor." Homocysteine is produced by eating "extreme-bad" proteins, like cooked meat and "bad proteins," like cooked fish and cheese below 50% fat. Deficiencies of vitamin B cause homocysteine to build up in the body.

Dr. Kilmer McCully, a pathologist at Harvard University and Massachusetts Hospital, linked homocysteine to vitamin B deficiency, 30 years ago.[30] But his research was ignored. Instead, federal money was poured into cholesterol research.

76

Dr. Thomas James, president of the American Heart Association during that period, said, "Pharmaceutical companies didn't want to fund homocysteine research because there was no money in the cure.[30] Most people with a high homocysteine level don't get enough folate (also called folic acid), vitamin B_6, or vitamin B_{12} in their diet. Replacing these vitamins by eating the right foods helps return the homocysteine level to normal.

Your body is a finely tuned BioChemical Machine. Keeping its complex chemical make-up balanced is the key to good health—not omitting certain foods from your diet, even those that contain saturated fat. If you always ate according to the perfect match of food chemistry and body chemistry, you would build up neither cholesterol nor homocysteine.

Plainly put, you need to increase the intake of base-builders, instead of lowering or omitting saturated fats. If you have already developed chronic diseases, you should avoid every food item that is marked by the color gray and red on the LEVEL TWO A&B Chart. However, you may eat all Neutral products, including butter, smoked fish, cured meat or rolled ham, salami, sour cream, cheese *above* 60% and many other food items. These are all products containing saturated fat, supposedly responsible for the increase in cholesterol and risk of heart disease, which is not the case.

If you have high cholesterol, you should place special emphasis on whole wheat products while avoiding unhealthy acid-builders such as white flour or white rice; balancing your diet between 80% base-builders *(yellow)* and 20% (healthy) acid-builders *(white)*.

The unsaturated fat-acids and rich fibers like cellulose and hemicellulose in these foods lower the cholesterol in the blood. And fiber binds cholesterol.

Also, you should studiously avoid trans fat, the unnatural and highly processed fat that is cheaply manufactured for use in restaurants to fry things like French fries.

After four weeks, your cholesterol will be significantly reduced, blood circulation will improve, and, the risk of arteriosclerosis will be minimized. These are all just some of side benefits of following the A&B principles.

Chapter 8

FAD DIETS:
Why Some of Them "Work" Temporarily!

Dieting has become a national obsession and made losing weight big business. Yet, despite all the diet pills, slimming drinks, diet products, and new guru inventions, obesity in Americans is reaching epidemic proportions. Warnings from nutrition and health experts about the pointlessness of serial dieting have had little impact. Millions of dieters continue to torture themselves; and in the end for nothing because diets don't work. Ninety percent of dieters gain all the weight back.

But why are some guru diets successful in the short run? After studying countless books from so called diet "experts," I came to realize that their hook is basically deprivation. Every guru instructs you to omit significant food groups from your day-to-day diet.

One vilifies dairy products; another, carbohydrates; and others, proteins in their entirety. Or fat, oil, saturated fat and cholesterol are the "main villain." And if it's no longer cholesterol and saturated fat, well, then they'll find another scapegoat, like casein,* to become the root of all evil.

Once they've got you hooked, fad diets sell you on the idea that you need "urgent" cleansing. But many of these detoxification programs are based primarily on a lot of "bad" or "extreme-bad" protein and almost all require giving up certain food groups. In short, they are based on a type of starvation.** Gurus "prescribe" these high protein diets – heavily promoted today as low carb diets - because it is the easiest way for them to make money.

Over-eating "extreme-bad" protein is not what your metabolism requires. Your body needs base-forming foods—alkalinity—to counteract the acid debris released into the circulation when cells die. If we eat too much protein and too little carbohydrates and fat, the body is forced to obtain its energy from protein, especially the "extreme-bad" protein that is only an emergency supplier to our metabolism. Remember Step #2 from the Big Seven Essentials? Eating too much "extreme-bad" protein drains your alkaline reserve and your Bio-Chemical Machine suffers.

---

*Casein is present in milk as calcium-salt and creates the milky color. It is the main protein of milk, from which it can be separated by the action of acid, the enzyme rennin, or bacteria (souring). Milk contains amino acids and phosphoric acids. Phosphate salts or ester of phosphoric acid is involved in many biochemical processes, often as part of complex molecules.
**Acidosis is a very prominent condition in starvation. When base-forming foods are withheld from the digestive tract, there is nothing to tie or bind the acids and we get the acid build-up found in starvation.

Why Do Bad Fad Diets Persist?

People continue to buy into fad diets because of short-term results—results that come from eliminating major food groups from their diet.

But let's face it; nobody can go forever without bread, macaroni (especially macaroni and cheese), potatoes, rice, noodles, pasta and pizza. Right? Healthy carbohydrates (from Groups I and II) are our body's number two energy supplier, especially after 50. More to the point, we love eating them!

Yet thirty years after I tried (without success) the dangerous high-protein diets myself, I couldn't believe what was happening: the ("extreme-bad") protein diet from the 1960s was back. Why? The answer is simple but significant. With high protein diets, you eat foods like those from the "B"-column, foods like those from the Neutral column, but *completely eliminate carbohydrates from the "A"-column.*

That's why unhealthy high-protein diets (today promoted as low-carb diets) work for a while—because by eating a lot of cooked meats, you are eating *partially* according to the A&B principles.

Unfortunately, once you resume your normal eating habits—not only eating meat and fat but also eating bread, macaroni, potatoes, rice, noodles, pasta, and pizza—you can't keep the pounds off.

Then there's another popular diet that is the exact opposite, dictating that you should eat only carbohydrates with some foods from the Neutral column and completely eliminate proteins from your diet.

Again, you are eating partially according to the A&B principles; and again, that's why it works for a while. So you can eat whole wheat bread, potatoes, couscous, brown rice, and whole wheat noodles, with vegetables, salads and fruits but you are not allowed to eat fat, Neutral meat, fish, and milk and other vital dairy products. If you like milk and dairy products, well, then, you are, according to these gurus, "suckling a cow." Of course, there is no distinction between "good," "bad," and "extreme-bad" p r o t e i n s o r t h e tremendous importance of milk to our health.

The Confusion Gurus Created by Distorting Hay's Original Research

The problem with most diet programs is that gurus have purposely dissected Dr. Hay's original research, taking a little from here, a little from there to cobble together diets that have more to do with marketing than your health. From scientifically sound research on how to maintain a proper acid-alkaline balance, they oversimplified Dr. Hay's work to invent a fashionable—and completely misleading—new concept: food combining.

Eating carbohydrates and proteins at the same time is our nature. The A&B Method is about dealing with historically new food items—food items that played no role in the development of our body's chemistry. In the framework of the A&B principles, all food items are classified according to the perfect match with our body's chemistry.

You will find vegetables in three different groups; fruits in three different groups; dairy products in two different groups; meat, fish, and nuts in three different groups. Even the egg is divided in two different groups.

Diet gurus, on the other hand, classify meat, fish, eggs and dairy products in one group only: "proteins." This is wrong. Matching food chemistry with body chemistry is just not that simple. This is why these food-combining gurus omit significant food groups as a whole and don't even separate the correct food items.

I read food-combining diet books (all based on separating carbohydrates from proteins) that advise their readers to eat pasta with tomato sauce, assuming that pasta was a concentrated carbohydrate and that tomato was a vegetable, thus Neutral. This information is all wrong. It is correct that raw tomatoes are vegetables, thus Neutral. But, once tomatoes have been cooked, they turn into an acid-building "B"-food item.

Also, the Neutrals, such as nuts, seeds, sour cream, mayonnaise, oil, butter, and whipped and heavy cream had become, miraculously, proteins that may not be combined with carbohydrates. Fruits from the "B"-column, such as apples, peaches, oranges, pineapples, strawberries, along with the Neutral vegetables have been reborn as carbohydrates. Other gurus advise you to eat rice with pineapples; tofu with honey; wheat with lemon. This is all incomprehensible nonsense.

The A&B Method is NOT about separating or eliminating foods. If you follow the distorted advice of diet gurus, than you go on and on unknowingly eating incompatible food, never ridding your body of toxins and then wonder why losing weight is so difficult.

Fad diets don't work because they do not eliminate the cause of obesity, fatigue and disease: self-poisoning.

You can torture yourself for a few weeks, following their strict regimens, being unbearably hungry, but you'll probably join the 90% of dieters who eventually lapse back into their old ways.

Even if you muster enough willpower to follow a strict diet regimen, the day will come when you'll find yourself unable to lose any more weight. *The laws of body chemistry upset your fad diet and suddenly you are stuck!* And remember the yo-yo effect: the more diets you try, the less you will be able to lose weight.

All fad diets are stressful, but they also trigger hazards to your health.

"Most such [fad] diets . . . are ineffective and sometimes much worse . . . and could put heart patients at risk in the long-term. Short-term success adds to the diets' allure. Some fad diets induce temporary weight loss just by restricting calories or imposing a monotony that kills the appetite. Others bring about water loss with their high-fat, low carbohydrate content.

"But extreme dieting can pose dangers. The fast fat-burning caused by drastic diets releases ketones, or acids, into the blood, in a process called ketosis. Excess ketosis can damage your health and can even put dieters with diabetes into a coma."

—Marilyn Chase, "Health Journal," *The Wall Street Journal* (April 7, 1997, page B1)

Chase is right. Most fad diets require starving, and starvation causes acidosis.

You will not only have difficulty losing weight, because you are starving, but also you will be poisoning your cells, i.e., yourself.

"Ketogenic diets cause a loss of body water, sodium and potassium. Dieters can experience dizziness, or elevated uric acid putting them at risk for kidney stones and gout. At worst, an electrolyte imbalance from mineral loss can trigger heart-rhythm disturbances. We've had people [who] passed out after losing too many minerals."
—Ellen Coleman, a dietitian in Riverside, California, quoted in the "Health Journal" section of *The Wall Street Journal*, April 7, 1997

Without knowledge of the match of food chemistry and body chemistry there is no such thing as a lasting solution, regardless of what you have been promised. As we grow older, the struggle to lose weight through fad diets only grows more difficult. Remember the law of our body chemistry: beginning at age thirty, cell activity begins to slow down more and more with each passing decade.

Healthy eating is possible, even in our modern world, if we apply a new way of thinking about food. Creating the perfect match between food chemistry and body chemistry is a way of life—not a temporary fix.

Chapter 9

TRUE OR FALSE
Can Tofu Fight Cancer?

If your doctor tells you that you have cancer, you feel as if a jury has convicted you for a crime you didn't commit. Because of its insidious nature, cancer is not an illness that can be treated with a 100% predictable outcome. I remember how devastated I was when I found out that I had cancer and would be losing my kidneys. I know how it feels to be desperately looking for something that can save your life. Reaching for every hope, every straw, every illusion is better than just looking forward, helplessly, to getting sicker and sicker until the day you die.

So I can truly understand how a simple food item, such as tofu, could be set up as having almost magical anti-cancer properties. "Like other beans, soybeans contain the anti-cancer compounds protease inhibitors," writes the diet-author, Judy Lin Eftekar in her book, *Feed Yourself Right*.[32] "Researchers at Japan's National

Cancer Center noted that people who eat macrobiotic miso soup every day (a popular soup made from soybean paste) are 33% less likely to have stomach cancer...Substituting meat with soy products like tofu or texturized vegetable protein (TVP) has been shown to reduce the risk of breast cancer..."

Studies may seem to indicate that soy reduces the risk of cancer, but how can anyone know for certain? Statistics are not proof of cause and effect. Gurus have twisted the research about tofu to present it in a way that is misleading to people desperate to pin their hopes on something that might help them in their darkest hour.

This is not to say that tofu and its potential to deter cancer should be ignored. In the course of my research, I asked the renowned authority, Professor Claus Leitzmann to elaborate about tofu's beneficial qualities. "Tofu contains, besides many other substances, genistein (phytoestrogen*), which has anti-cancerogenic properties. The protein of the soybean is high-grade. The acid-basic actions are a question of the quantity of consumption."

---

*The phytoestrogens are divided into two groups: the Isaflavonoide and the Lignane. Famous Isoflavonoide are genistein and daidzein. These are found only in legumes (soybean, etc.) of the tropics. Traditional Asian nourishment consists of a multiple of isoflavonoiden by contrast to that of the American and European. As a result, the Asians are far less often afflicted with hormone-dependent conditions such as breast cancer. However, highly processed soybean products, such as soy sauce or tofu, do not contain the high levels of genistein found in unprocessed soybeans. As of this writing, isolation of phytoestrogen, such as genistein, has been unsuccessful. Therefore, equally effective phytoestrogens are not yet available to the consumer marked in a nourishment-supplement form. (Watzl, Bernhard; Leitzmann, Claus: *Bioactive Substances in Food*, Hippokrates Publ., 1999).

He also mentioned that "...East Asian people would profit from the consumption of tofu...yet, the isolation and application of the effective substances are problematic."

Too much has been made about the diets of Asian men and women and how their consumption of soy products might offer a form of cancer prevention. "Might," of course, is an important qualifier; there's no definitive proof. In addition, many tout that if most of your protein comes from "fat-free" soy products, then you can avoid beef and other high-fat meats.

Let's dispense with some of the misconceptions about soy. First of all, it is not fat-free. Soybeans contain 20% fat, the highest ratio among legumes. The soybean itself belongs to the legumes family, which includes beans, peas, and lentils. This means that soybeans, rich in protein, belong to the Neutral food group. Do you remember our slogan about Neutrals on the A&B Chart: *"24 hours a day, 7 days a week?"*

However, tofu, which contains 5 to 8% protein, 3 to 4% fat, 2 to 4% carbohydrates, and 0.6% minerals, is a *processed* food item, made of soymilk. Soymilk is made of soybeans, a healthy, base-building plant. However, in order to produce soymilk, soybeans are soaked for only 12 hours in 10 times the quantity of water. Beans, EVERY BEAN, needs to be soaked in water for many more hours in order to activate the chemical process which, ultimately, turns the beans into a healthy food item. Afterwards, the soaked soybeans are ground and heated to 100 degrees Celsius (212 degrees Fahrenheit) and centrifuged. During this process, the so-called soymilk emerges, from which they make tofu.[33]

The most damaging thing I have ever read from those spreading misleading messages about tofu was a book by a diet guru who refers openly to Dr. Hay's research. This guru, too, speaks of the acid-alkaline balance, yet the book was crowded with mistakes about chemistry. The real problem was that this guru recommended tofu as a base-builder, which is dangerous advice for someone battling a major disease. Base-builders, YELLOW on the A&B Chart, can and should be eaten every day as much as possible, which is not the case with tofu. Unfortunately, many cancer patients believe such advice, clinging to the hope that eating huge amounts of tofu can help overcome their disease.

To be honest, if I had cancer and I didn't know about the A&B Method, I would start eating tofu like crazy too, hoping that it would save me. It would intrigue me that Asians are famous for their health, and this might influence me to believe that there was, indeed, a yearned-for wonder antidote that just needed to be eaten. But this is not the case and not the reason diet gurus are "selling" their miraculous tofu diets to you.

First of all, Asians eat a little bit differently than the way described by gurus, who, obviously, discovered that Asian diets and alternative medicine are marketable. Secondly, lumping all Asians into one category is vague, since cultures and cuisine differ from country to country, from eating habits to eating habits, and from poor to rich. Which Asian population is the basis for tofu's cancer fighting properties—the Chinese, Japanese, Korean, Vietnamese, Tibetan, Philippine, or Taiwanese?

Let's take, for example, the Chinese, considered by many to be among the healthiest people on earth. Can their high standard of health be attributed to eating huge portions of tofu, miso, and other soy products? It's more likely that their primary diet of vegetables, salads, sprouts (the natural soybean is a strong base-builder), fruits and natural rice lends them the properties they need for good health. What's more, for the Chinese, cooked meat, fish, or (processed) tofu are delicacies—eaten only from time to time in addition to their basic foods.

One of the reasons the Chinese are in such good health is that their traditional eating habits mirror the A&B Method, inadvertently matching the chemistry of the foods they eat with their body chemistry. For example, rice is found in the "A"-column; vegetables, salads and tofu are Neutral. Chemically, that's the perfect combination. Even the famous Peking duck with oranges or nectarines naturally follows the A&B Chart. Meat is a strong acid-builder and "B"-fruits are strong base-builders, which neutralize the acid as long as no third-party foods from "A"-column join the digestion process. The truth is that Asian eating patterns are very much like that of our early ancestors.

China is at this time still a so-called developing country. These people are relatively poor; therefore, it is not unusual for a large family to consume meat like chicken, pork, or beef on only special occasions.

These habits echo those of our ancestors and are still very much the case in other Arabian and African countries where you'll find the oldest and healthiest people on earth. Reaching the age of 100 is not exceptional.

Yet, longevity has nothing to do with race. As Professor Claus Leitzman said, "The Caucasus people can reach the highest ages; over 100 years is common!" He's right. The secret to a long, healthy life lies in making sure the nourishment of our cells is chemically balanced.

Fortunately, in our western world, many progressive medical doctors include the eating habits of their patients in their recovery of disease, including cancer. If you are fighting disease, you should abide by the LEVEL TWO A&B Chart. If you look at the chart, you can see, tofu is a perfectly healthy, beneficial food when eaten the A&B way; which is to say eat as much from the YELLOW as possible, moderately of the WHITE (where you'll find tofu), and rarely, if at all from the RED & GRAY.

Eating according to the A&B Method is a vital way to bolster your immune system in its fight against disease. Don't be fooled into thinking one food, like tofu, can single-handedly solve your health problems. A comprehensive non-diet based on the A&B principles will enable your body to dedicate its full resources to getting better. Later chapters will talk about some of the specific foods you should be eating to optimize on your body's ability to heal. If you do so, I believe your body will react the same as mine did and continues to do.

PART IV

THE
MILK & APPLE
THERAPY

Chapter 10

THE TRUTH ABOUT MILK

The first food we eat when we come into the world is milk. Mother's milk is nature's perfect food. Mostly water, the remainder is made up of 6.9% carbohydrates, 3.7% fat, 1.2% protein, lactose, pantothenic acid, potassium, phosphorus, iron, and vitamin A, B_1, B_2, B_6, D, and C. As infants incapable of digesting regular food, milk is the ideal food for our developing BioChemical Machines. In a sense, infants "eat" milk, as it is the only source of their nourishment. As we get older, we no longer "eat" milk. Instead, we drink it. Now, it's no longer human milk, but cow's milk, ideally whole and organic. Due to its treatment, milk's composition has shifted to 3.4% protein, 3.4% fat, and 4.7% carbohydrates, but it's still good for us and we consume it with our breakfast, lunch, and dinner because we know it helps our bodies' calcium requirements.

As everyone knows, milk and milk products are loaded with calcium. What's more, one glass of whole milk (250 ml) contains only 8 grams of fat; a fragment of the total of 60 to 80 grams of fat that may be eaten over the course of a day by healthy, moderately active persons. In so many ways milk is, in a word, great.

- Calcium is important not only for healthy bones, but also for skin, hair, eyesight, cell growth, and thyroid gland functions.

- "A daily under-supply of 300 mg calcium means the loss of 10% bone-mass within one year," according to Professor Helmuth Minne, University of Heidelberg.

- "Without calcium, nerves and muscles cannot function, our heart wouldn't beat regularly, and the blood wouldn't clot," Professor Minne further states. "In order to make calcium accessible to your bones, you need vitamin D, which is also found in milk. Vitamin D is the key which opens the door to the bone for calcium to enter."[34]

- A study at the University of California at San Diego showed that people who drank milk were one-third less likely to develop colorectal cancer than those who didn't.[35]

- Another study at the University of California at San Diego showed that acidophilus milk, a fermented form of milk, is a deterrent against colon cancer.[35]

- In another research study at the University of California at San Diego, milk was linked to a decreased incidence of stomach and lung cancer. And the calcium in milk may help prevent intestinal cancer.[35]

- Non-milk drinkers are twice as likely to have high blood pressure as those who drink milk, according to a study of 8,000 men by the National Heart, Lung and Blood Institute.

- Through extensive research, scientists at the University of California at San Diego discovered that milk contains an amazing property besides calcium—an "unidentified factor" that has been shown to retard bone disease and control blood pressure.[35]

Despite so many scientifically established benefits, self-appointed diet "experts" have reviled milk and milk products for years. Unfortunately, many have brought into this nonsense. Although, the dairy industry has made the mistake of adding hormones, antibiotics, and chemicals to their products, today increasing numbers of dairy farmers are producing hormone-, antibiotic-, and pesticide-free whole milk. Ask for it! The more people ask, the more organic whole milk will become available..

But you may say that you can't drink milk because you're lactose intolerant. Well, you wouldn't be alone, but it's not a condition that should stand in your way of enjoying the benefits of milk.

Lactose Intolerance

"The milk of cows, goats and sheep is often consumed by humans, but only Western societies drink milk after infancy; for people in most of the world, milk causes flatulence and diarrhea," states *Webster's Encyclopedia.*[36] Two-thirds of the world's population gets sick from drinking milk because they lack the enzyme to digest cow's milk—otherwise known as lactose intolerance.

But why is this so, if milk is so healthy? The answer is in the way we consume milk. To do so in a healthy way requires knowledge about the match of the food chemistry with the chemistry of the body.

I was captivated with the insight that "only Western societies drink milk after infancy." The Bedouins in Arabia and North Africa and others who retained the eating habits of their ancestors won't *drink* cow, goat, or sheep milk. Instead, milk is processed into yogurt, sour milk, Kefir, and cheese, all of which are Neutral food items. Only infants drink milk. For adults, goat or camel milk is eaten in the forms described above; usually as a complete meal in which they don't add other foods. Here's where the Western world encounters its problem with milk. We usually consume milk with the wrong foods, like cereal, bread, potatoes, rice, or pasta. Remember, processed milk products such as yogurt, heavy cream, sour milk, whey, and cream cheese are Neutral and can be eaten with cereal, bread, potatoes, rice, pasta and sugar products—but not with the liquid form of milk, which if you refer to the A&B Chart, can be found in the "B"-column.

We have to understand that homogenizing and pasteurizing interferes with nature. Original whole milk was (before being homogenized and pasteurized) a strong base-builder, belonging to the Neutrals and therefore easy to digest and very healthy. It could be eaten with anything, including cereal, bread, potatoes, rice, or pasta. But this doesn't apply to the milk we buy in supermarkets today which has been changed through the industrial process. Yet, despite the processing of milk, it remains a moderate base-builder with its healthy vitamins A, D, B_2, B_{12}, H, and minerals intact, as well as the "unidentified factor" that researchers discovered.

So how can we capitalize on the healthy aspects of milk? The answer is simple—"eat" milk with base-forming foods, such as apples, pineapples, oranges, melons, and other exotic fruits from the "B"-column and, of course, Neutral groups, especially Neutral cheeses. Due to its detoxifying effect on our system, it is an excellent idea to consume whole milk in the morning with other strong base-builders, especially apples, which I'll talk about more in later chapters. Avoid consuming milk with foods from the "A"-columns like bananas, raisins, grapes, figs, and dates.

> *BioChemical Machine Fact: It's very important to keep in mind that you may go through a so-called HEALING PROCESS, an adjustment period while the body works hard to get rid of the poison.*

For approximately one week you **might** experience diarrhea, headaches, and shooting pains. This adjudtment can differs based on age or current state of health.

This HEALING PROCESS can be and often is mistaken for LACTOSE INTOLERANCE due to a similarity of symptoms!

Don't worry. Just stick to the A&B principles; soon, you'll be amazed that you can drink milk without experiencing any discomfort.

BioChemical Machine Fact: *There are some RARE cases of people who suffer from MILK-PROTEIN ALLERGY. They must avoid dairy products or eat them according to their physician's advice.*

The most important calcium suppliers are milk and milk products. Many vegetables and herbs, such as parsley, chives, and dill, offer relatively high calcium content; however, the body cannot utilize them as easily as milk and milk products. If you are still reluctant to drink milk, you can still reap its benefits by consuming other dairy products from the Neutral group, such as yogurt, buttermilk, whey or Kefir, cream, sour cream, cottage cheese, cream cheese, or goat's milk cheese.

BioChemical Machine Fact: *In addition to the other benefits, YOGURT counteracts the bacteria that cause urinary infection.*

The most impressive quality of milk may be the relief it can provide for the 38 million Americans who suffer from arthritis[37] or osteoporosis. I am one of them. For many years, I refused to drink milk because of the chemicals, hormones, antibiotics, and pesticides that were added.

However, when I became crippled by rheumatoid arthritis, I began following a diet based on 80% base-builders and only 20% acid-builders. This change in my eating habits included consuming milk along with peaches and oranges at which point, I made a revolutionary discovery, the story of which I would like to share with you in the next chapter.

Chapter 11

ARTHRITIS & A TRUE
MIRACLE DRUG

Unfortunately, we often don't follow good advice until problems arise. And so it was with my milk consumption. Put off by its chemicals and hormones, I avoided drinking milk every day. For fifteen years, I followed the basic A&B principles and felt great.

I overlooked that by age thirty, cell activity begins to slow down, a decline that only accelerates as we get older. I just felt too good. I didn't think about taking preventive steps to address this change; namely eating 80% base-builders and only 20% acid-builders as was recommended in Dr. Hay's original work. Also, I wasn't avoiding "bad" and "extreme-bad" proteins, which you should do, especially after surgery. In fact, I indulged in a lot of "bad" and "extreme-bad" proteins. Why would I take such a chance with my health? I didn't know any better! *Because the discovery had yet to be made!*

It would be much later, with the help of Professor Luke Burke, PhD, Chairman of the Department of Chemistry at Rutgers University, that I would expand on Dr. Hay's original work and make my most important discovery: that there is a vast chemical difference between "good," "bad," and "extreme—bad" proteins. These revolutionary findings would ultimately help me develop LEVEL TWO of the A&B Chart.

As I look back now, I realize that it was a personal crisis that forced me to dig deeper into Dr. Hay's research, looking for answers in his work for an affliction that was making my life a living hell: arthritis. At that time, I didn't know that lurking around the corner was an ailment that could make life miserable. I never wondered about brittle bones or a crippled body. In my mind, arthritis was something for "old people." Certainly not for me, although I was no longer what we call young. In those days I felt even better and more energetic than when I was in my 20s. Being in great shape, I never imagined that a terrible disease would attack my bones.

Yet, one day, pains gradually began in my left thumb. I ignored the pain. I wanted to believe that it was an injury, perhaps caused while training our frisky dog. Soon after, I began to experience increasing pain in my spine, but again, I dismissed it as probably the result of an old riding accident. But over the following months, the pain in my thumb increased. After a while, I couldn't even hold a cup anymore. The pain started to keep me awake at nights. After a couple of months my thumb became crooked. I was shocked and I tried to straighten it by using force.

After the suffering spread to my feet, legs, knees, hips, and shoulders, I finally went to a doctor who told me I had rheumatoid arthritis. He could do no more for me than prescribe painkillers and calcium, which did little to alleviate my pain. Gradually, the agony worsened to the point that I could no longer get up without the help of a cane.

I panicked. But being a researcher, I quickly realized my energy was better spent collecting information. In the course of my research, I kept coming back to the fact that milk can cure some bone problems and possesses the ability to detoxify the body. I guess it was out of desperation that I remembered Hay's teachings about the acid-alkaline balance/reserve and the vital ratio of 80% base-builders and 20% acid-builders. Yet, at that time I didn't know that there was a vast difference between the healthy acid-builders and the unhealthy ones! Or rather, those that you can now find shaded WHITE on the LEVEL TWO A&B Chart (the healthy acid-builders) and those that are really bad—the GRAY and the RED.

The next morning I drank three glasses of whole milk and ate peaches. Of course, I didn't drink low-fat or fat-free milk since I knew that the dairy industry puts sugar and chemicals in low or non-fat products to make them taste better or more like whole milk. I took the whole milk like medicine. But my unprepared body reacted adversely to the milk, as if I had drunk camel's milk or castor oil. I called my reaction "races to the bathroom."

I didn't know it at the time, but I would later discover that my body's reaction to the milk was a healing process—a normal, temporary period of adjustment in which the body's chemistry corrects and cleanses itself.

Later, as I began to test my theories on others, both my personal "guinea pigs" and later, on test subjects at a private clinic, I discovered that *people were confusing this healing process with lactose intolerance.* From then on I started my day with whole milk and foods that strictly adhered to the 80% base-builders and not more than 20% acid-builders rule. But the pain didn't really go away.

At that time I lived in a beautiful farm area in New Jersey that was ideal for a researcher. The only things that could interrupt my thinking process were raccoons and rabbits. Since they didn't bother me (instead, my beloved dogs bothered them), I was focused on my increasing and frightening pain.

It was pure chance that my neighbor, the owner of an apple farm in this area, visited me one evening and brought a gift of a huge bag filled with big green Granny Smith apples. It was also pure chance that I ate, next morning, two of these apples together with my "medicine," the milk. Why? I hadn't shopped for a week and my refrigerator was almost empty. There wasn't anything else but milk and apples available.

I was surprised to find that after drinking only one glass of milk (250 ml) and eating two apples, I felt like I had eaten a big, satisfying breakfast! The hunger that usually plagued me by mid-morning never materialized.

Furthermore, by the next day, I realized that my pain had lessened! I showed my husband my previously bandaged and stiff thumb, which I now could move.

Gradually, the pain vanished throughout my body. After two weeks of this new "cure," my thumb was flexible. I was, of course, thrilled, and completely dedicated to sticking to this new powerhouse union of apples and milk. In the course of my recovery, I became curious. I wanted to uncover the reason behind this amazing discovery.

I knew that the main supplier for energy, besides carbohydrates, is (healthy) fat. For years I had primarily eaten olive oil and butter. But I wanted to find out whether or not the "fat-free," "low-fat" and "2 % fat" milk, combined with apples, would have the same effect as the whole milk. It didn't work. Soon after breakfast, I was very hungry and even felt mild pain in some parts of my body. The reaction of my body was only logical since sugar added to these other kinds of milk, is a strong acid builder. Besides that, I violated the A&B principles. Apples belong to the food in the "B"-column and sugar to "A"-column. Still, I was very surprised by my body's almost immediate reaction.

It really hit me when I focused on the fact that after drinking whole milk and eating the apples in the morning, I would not be hungry for hours to come. I was totally fascinated by these results. What was it that was so powerful? After a couple of days and a lot of pondering, I realized: *two powerful base-builders are joining forces*. That means, your metabolism gets it all: pure vitamins and minerals.

These discoveries captured my scholarly heart. I couldn't resist asking my mother to be my guinea pig since she suffered from lactose intolerance and osteoporosis. She, as many others, grew up with old-fashioned and wrong ideas about eating. I was convinced that she might have developed lactose intolerance over the course of several decades, especially since she didn't have this problem when I was a child. I wondered, perhaps if self-poisoning was responsible for the disappearance of the appropriate enzyme required to digest milk? I wanted to determine whether or not my mother could detoxify her body with the A&B principles as I had done. If so, she could start drinking milk, which would help her osteoporosis, without having to experience the nasty side-effects of lactose intolerance.

My mother followed the A&B teachings and ate precisely the foods that her body needed. She ate moderate quantities of Neutral dairy products or whole milk with apples or other "B"-fruits, salads and/or vegetables. One of the first things she reported was that she enjoyed drinking milk for the first time in years, especially with apples; the unpleasant mucous build-up she had always associated with milk disappeared. She also reported feeling more rejuvenated than she had in years. Significantly, we discovered that it was NOT the milk alone that caused her lactose intolerance. Once her body chemistry was balanced, she could cope with milk again; the symptoms of lactose intolerance disappeared.

Her skeleton now benefits from the high calcium content of the whole milk. And the pain she felt from osteoporosis, which has stopped progressing, went away completely.

Two-thirds of the population in western countries are lactose intolerant. If the Milk & Apple Therapy can have the same impact on others that it had on my mother, than these findings are significant. It would demonstrate that lactose intolerance is, in most cases, nothing but the so-called healing process.

I couldn't resist recruiting friends to participate in my experiment.

The result was overwhelming. Everybody who followed the Milk and Apple Therapy and the A&B Method was soon able to drink and enjoy whole milk. One of my test subjects wrote me the following enthusiastic letter on August 19, 1998:

...By the way, the new eating plan that you gave us is not only easy to follow, but it has also given us a lot more energy! In addition to this, I might add, that we have begun to eat an apple with a glass of milk at the start of each day...like you had suggested. I thought you might also like to know that prior to this, I was unable to drink whole milk, as I was lactose intolerant. However, when I drink the whole milk while eating the apple, I have no negative reactions. I feel healthy and I believe you are right about the cleansing benefits the two of these foods have for the body when eaten together.

As I said, these are not the only cases in the world that testify to the effectiveness of the A&B principles. There are millions of people in Arabia and Africa who still follow our species' original eating habits. They do not suffer from lactose intolerance, arthritis and osteoporosis.

But, interestingly enough, wealthy people in Arabia and Africa suffer from the same diseases as we do; no doubt, because they have adapted to our eating habits.

Only two years after having discovered the Milk & Apple Therapy, I had forgotten the unbearable pain caused by arthritis. I asked myself, 'what would happen if I returned to my bad old eating habits?' I had become curious. My scholarly heart was challenged and I couldn't resist trying "the old way."

I stopped drinking whole milk and eating apples in the morning. I ate little of potatoes, raw vegetables, salads and fruits, and increased the amount of cooked meat I consumed. I also ate packaged snack foods: cheese curls, barbecued potato chips and other junk food.

After a short period of time, mild pain in my hands, joints, and hips began to bother me. I was extremely tired. I experienced increasing pain in my left kidney. After five weeks, the pain in my bones, especially hip, increased dramatically. I needed the help of a cane to get up from the couch and walk. I did what I hadn't done in years; I took heavy painkillers. But the pain didn't stop. My hips and spine ached as badly as they had after a long-ago, serious riding accident.

I didn't wait long before I went, in tremendous pain and almost in tears, to a nearby supermarket to buy all kinds of food that increase the body's alkalinity: cauliflower, broccoli, carrots, spinach, white and red cabbage, sprouts, onions, parsley, chives, all kind of lettuce—and a lot of potatoes. I prepared a huge bowl of salad, consisting of lettuce and vegetables, olive oil, apple vinegar, sea salt and steamed potatoes with skins.

I anxiously temporized the waiting period of three hours in order to drink (late in the night) my "medicine": three glasses of whole milk (each glass 250 ml) and two apples. Soon, the pain lessened, and within a couple of days I was almost back on track. After two weeks, I was completely pain-free.

I intentionally repeated this self-experiment four more times. After a period of feeling well and fit and healthy, I would dabble with eating the "old way." Every time the results were the same: pain, lack of energy, and more pain.

After these four times, I decided to leave the clinical tests to clinical researchers and their subjects. I had the proof I needed. Now I knew that this experiment could be done with every person under clinical scientific supervision. Ultimately, the accuracy of my findings were confirmed.

After having experienced, personally, such over-whelming results, there was no doubt in my mind that whole milk and apples are a true miracle drug. From then on, I tried to convince everyone who was experiencing pain to convert their eating habits to the A&B Method and at least give the Milk & Apple Therapy a try.

Despite my good intentions, I often faced tremendous skepticism. "Try it at least for a couple of days," I would urge, "you have nothing to lose, and so much to gain!" Only those who were already seriously ill and full of pain followed my advice. I managed to convince my husband—a true skeptic. When the pain of his arthritis became so bad that he could hardly climb the stairs in our house, he decided it couldn't hurt to at least try the A&B Method and Milk & Apple Therapy.

After a short period of time, he had the same results as everyone else.

Others found a breakfast consisting of milk and apples, simply bizarre. "Why would this have such a profound effect on my well-being?" was the most common question I heard. I never got tired of explaining to people the reason behind the Milk & Apple Therapy's effectiveness: *Two base-builders join forces.* Apples, a strong base-builder, support the unique effects of milk, which, even in its treated (pasteurized) form, remains a moderate base-builder.

And I referred again and again to the scientific studies conducted at the University of California at San Diego supporting the *unidentified factor in milk* that is so beneficial to our health.

I pondered to myself: "What exactly is the secret behind milk and apples?" I found the answer by taking the example of a baby. If a baby vomits mother-milk, the milk comes out already "curdled" through the stomach's acidity. The same is true for milk products that have been made sour. This curdling is a fermentation process caused through enzymatic lactic acid that prepares food for digestion.

This example opened my eyes to the logic behind milk and apple's success. "B"-fruits are not only strong base-builders, but also contain fruit-acid (a short-term acid supply). In short, milk and "B"-fruits are a symbiosis that promotes the digestion. The simultaneous delivery of alkalinity by two powerful base-builders—and the effectiveness with which it can detoxify the body—is the reason why milk and apples could cure my arthritis, my mother's lactose intolerance, and my husband's arthritis. They all swear by this true miracle "therapy" and wouldn't change their breakfast for anything in this world.

I was determined to convince people that this approach to food was the smart way to balance out our interference with nature. One of those whom I converted to my cause is a 55-year-old American worker. On May 25, 1998, after only two weeks of following the A&B Method, he wrote the following letter:

In 1991 I was working as a warehouse person in New Jersey. While unloading a truck of padding for wall-to-wall carpet, I twisted my back, causing me to leave work for almost two weeks.

When I returned to work, my back was never the same. I eventually left work and applied for workers compensation... In August of 1994 I was diagnosed with osteo-arthritis. I saw doctors at Metropolitan Hospital's Orthopedic Department in New York City and also spoke with Orthopedic Surgeons at Albany Medical Center, Albany, New York. The diagnosis was firm...I couldn't work, run, lift heavy objects, climb stairs without effort, or play with my children. I was placed on anti-inflammatory drugs (non steroidal), and pain medication was prescribed. I was told not to do anything high impact that could cause further injury to my hips.

In May of 1998, I had the good fortune of meeting Eleonora De Lennart through my wife. De Lennart learned that I had osteoarthritis and asked to meet me. With reluctance I went to her home and spoke with her. She asked me all kinds of questions.

All I thought of was "how much is this consultation going to cost?" She told me that she also was arthritic to the point that [she had] some deformity in her fingers. I said to myself "yeah, right." De Lennart told me that if I changed my eating habits I could possibly go back to a normal life...Although I've just started trying what she has advised, the results are amazing. I have a low tolerance for milk, so using plain yogurt and apples I decided to give it a try. On Monday, May 11, 1998, I started my day with two eight (8) ounce glasses of blended plain yogurt and two delicious apples.

I felt like I had eaten a whole breakfast, which I never do. I had to sit down and relax because I was so full.

After following her recommendations, about eight days later I had a burst of energy and decided to try to work in the yard raking leaves and pruning some trees and bushes. I put in about five hours of yard work which I haven't done in the past four years. The thing I noticed most was I didn't seem to have a need for my pain medication which I usually take after any physical exertion. I still took my anti-inflammatories. The daily pain I had been experiencing decreased a lot. I also made mention to my wife that I felt pretty good after doing that work. I don't know what the process is, but I do know that I'm not walking with much of a gait anymore, I can walk up stairs with less effort, and the range of motion concerning my hips has greatly improved. I know different things work for different people, but I firmly believe that meeting Eleonora De Lennart has changed my life.

She's shown me how to change my eating habits and because of this, though I'm not 100%, I'm 65% and getting better...

Since then, he exchanged the yogurt with milk and is recovering dramatically. Recently he paid me a visit. He literally came dancing into my house. Shouting, "I love you! I love you! You changed my life!"

You may question the dramatic results of following the A&B Method, but EVERYBODY in my experiments has had similar results. Even if you're a skeptic, you have nothing to lose by at least trying the A&B Method of approaching food, especially if you're suffering from pain or disease. Within a very short period of time, you'll have all the evidence you need.

The Milk & Apple Therapy is an easy-to-follow treatment that, obviously, anyone can initiate at home, Nonetheless, it is based on scientifically sound research. Over 28 million Americans suffer from arthritis.

The research data currently available should be further developed so that even advanced cases of arthritis and osteoporosis can profit from it.

Chapter 12

THE MILK & APPLE THERAPY
Uniting Two Food Powerhouses

Having personally experienced and witnessed such success with the milk and apple therapy, I wanted to find out why bringing these two foods together have such a powerful effect on our BioChemical Machine.

I was well aware of the beneficial qualities of milk—its high calcium content, many essential vitamins and minerals, as well as the "unidentified factor" that researchers had established could retard bone disease and control blood pressure.[51] But what was so special about apples? Although every fruit is extremely healthy, it became obvious that there is something about the chemical makeup of an apple that made it a powerhouse fruit.

I confided my ideas to a colleague who was a great proponent of the A&B Method, having experienced first hand the way it relieved his arthritis and high blood pressure, and the almost miraculous effect it had had on his mother's health.*

He suggested that there might be a correlation between the renowned health of Syrians and the Lebanese and their habit of eating apples. He pointed out that these people were legendary in the Arab world for their strong bones and living to an extremely old age, free of arthritis, heart, liver and kidney diseases.

I investigated and found that apples are indeed a major part of the Lebanese and Syrian diet, with which they eat, like most Arabs, healthy wheat bread, Neutral cheeses, vegetables, salads, olives, and other fruits. If they eat cooked meat it is only for special occasions and usually entails the preparation of a whole ox for a large group of people.

I was intrigued. Everyone knows the old saying, "An apple a day keeps the doctor away." I decided that I wanted to prove it. So I studied and analyzed the chemistry of apples, employing the help of food chemists like Hilka de Groot-Boehlhoff.[38] The result of my research was fascinating. I found that apples are the fruit equivalent of a jack-of-all trades:

- Apples are a strong base-building food, supplying the body with many essential enzymes, vitamins, and minerals.

- Apples stimulate metabolism and metabolize fat.

---

*At the beginning of July 1997, his 77-year-old mother was brought into the intensive care unit of a hospital because of dangerously high blood pressure, arteriosclerosis, high blood cholesterol, and calcification of coronary artery vessels. A blood clot in her artery had become life threatening and she was scheduled for surgery on July 16. My colleague insisted on feeding the A&B. The result: the surgery scheduled for July 16 was postponed. On July 29, 1997, the surgery was canceled and she checked out of the hospital.

- One-fourth of an apple's composition is a substance called *pectin*, which offers the body many healthful benefits:

- Pectin aids digestion.

- Pectin may help reduce cancer and heart disease.

- Pectin is a soluble fiber that lowers artery-clogging LDL blood cholesterol levels by reducing fat absorption.

- Pectin raises levels of HDL, the good cholesterol.

- Apples regulate the functioning of the intestine and relieve diarrhea.

- Apples are high in fiber, the "roughage" that keeps things moving smoothly through your digestive tract.

- Apples help keep blood sugar levels steady for long periods of time; good news for diabetics, hypoglycemics, and others who are sensitive to blood sugar highs and lows.

- Apples are loaded with boron, an essential trace element that helps harden bones.

- A Yale University study showed that apples lowered patients' blood pressure and the level of damaging cholesterol valances, as well as protected the heart and blood vessels.[39]

> **BioChemical Machine Fact**: *One medium apple contains 9 to 10 grams of fiber, a good portion of the 20 to 35 grams you need every day.*

A powerful agent in detoxifying cells, apples also help decompose acid deposits in the tissue—as does whole milk. Whole milk and apples are base-builders. Not only do they help rid the body of poison, but also they build up your alkalinity. They're the perfect food marriage: Apples metabolize the fat in whole milk, freeing milk's calcium to do its job. Then, your body can efficiently utilize its vitamins and minerals, and your alkaline savings account goes up.

What's more a well-balanced blood sugar level—which the apple helps to maintain—naturally curbs your appetite. Eating milk and apples in the morning staves off hunger for hours, no small consideration when trying to lose weight. Even though our culture is fixated on eating cereals, bread, bagels, and other carbohydrates in the morning, apples and whole milk are a far better breakfast choice. They help build a strong alkaline foundation for the day. Grain carbohydrates, according to our liver's rhythm, should be reserved for the afternoon and evening.

> **BioChemical Machine Fact:** *People with arthritis or osteoarthritis should drink at least one to two glasses of whole milk and eat at the least two large apples, such as Granny Smith, Empire, Golden Delicious, or McIntosh.*

As we know from the previous chapter, whole milk's high calcium protects against osteoporosis if you start drinking it early in life.

> **BioChemical Machine Fact:** *Research shows that most people get less than half the calcium they need every day. The Osteoporosis Foundation encourages drinking three glasses of milk a day to keep the bones in shape.*[40]

Continuing to get enough calcium is important throughout your life, because calcium is regularly drawn from your bones to perform jobs elsewhere in your body and then expelled from the body through urine and perspiration. Calcium must continually be replaced through food.*

Bones are a network of collagen fibers that are impregnated with inorganic salts, especially calcium phosphate. Enveloped within this solid matrix are bone cells, blood vessels, and nerves. The strength of the toughest bone is comparable to reinforced concrete. We need strong bones for overall strength and fitness. Supple bones also help prevent osteoporosis, a disease suffered mostly by women but also noted in men, in which weak bones become brittle with age.

Experiments have confirmed that eating cooked meat—the "extreme-bad" protein—causes high amounts of calcium to be expelled from the body. Over time, the consumption of "bad" protein causes over-acidification that can lead to a dismantling of bone substance.

---

*Scientists believe getting calcium from milk is better than calcium supplements.

If the body cannot buffer the acid in the blood, it is forced to mobilize calcium, magnesium and potassium from its reserves to balance the bases and acids. *And the reserves are in the skeleton.* The skeleton can be demineralized over the decades, and the bone will decalcify.

You can avoid acid formation by consuming whole milk and "B"-fruits, especially apples, along with calcium-forming foods and base-forming salads, vegetables and fruits.

You may be surprised to find fruits such as apples, pineapples, apricots, cherries and oranges, in the "B"-column, especially since all fruits are not only very healthy but also vital base-builders (yellow). Placing them in the "B"-column is a precaution: these particular fruits contain a short-term (healthy) acid supply and shouldn't be eaten with "A" foods at the same time.

PLEASE NOTE: People with chronic diseases should discuss the Milk & Apple Therapy with their medical doctor. Your doctor will be glad to help you to find out what's right for you.

All others should decide individually how much whole milk they would like to drink. But you should always eat two (or even more) apples, because this is one of the best things you can do for your body's savings account, the alkaline reserve.

PART V

IMPORTANT SPECIFICS

Chapter 13

SOME IMPORTANT SPECIFICS
About Losing Weight

The A&B Method is NOT a diet. If you follow the A&B Method, you will never be hungry while in the process of losing weight. Weight loss is just a side effect of balancing your body chemistry. With the A&B Method you don't need to torture yourself through a strict regimen and you don't have to be a part of the 90% of dieters who lapse back into their old ways. Remember the "yo-yo" effect. The more diets you try, the less likely you will be to lose weight.

The A&B Method is a permanent lifestyle adjustment that is easy to follow and very healthy. However, as is true with any change to your way of life, there are some specifics that you need know to keep you on track:

- The more you weigh when you start the A&B Method, the faster you'll shed pounds.

- After your initial success, your weight will plateau—it will seem like you're stuck, at least on the scale. Don't be fooled. Your body is in the process of being returned to its natural state of chemical balance. Just keep following the A&B Method.

- During this time, as your body works hard to get rid of toxins, don't eat chemically incompatible food (yes, I'm talking about a Big Mac). Allow your body at least six weeks to cleanse itself before giving into temptation.

- Don't be concerned if the weight you initially lose isn't concentrated on the areas of your body that you would like it to be. If you stick to the A&B Method, you will eventually lose weight all you're your body: face, hands, abdomen, thighs, and legs.

- Don't stress. It takes time for your body to get rid of its poison and for your weight to return to its ideal state. Avoid weighing yourself everyday. As you regain your good heath, you will experience phases that won't be evident on a scale.

> **(Fun!) BioChemical Machine Fact:**
> *After approximately four weeks of following the A&B*
> *Method, try slipping on an old pair of jeans that no*
> *longer fit. They may still be tight, but you will find that,*
> *perhaps, you can close the zipper—an exciting*
> *milestone on the road to losing weight.*

There are variables to how quickly you will shed excess pounds: your age, personal constitution and level of activity. If you are not older than age 35, then 20 to 25 pounds in six weeks is not impossible. But I urge you to take your time as you follow the A&B Method, especially at the beginning.

Later, when you have detoxified your body, your acid-alkaline balance is restored, and you have lost the weight you wanted to lose, it's possible, even likely, that you'll backslide into your old bad eating habits. If that happens, don't worry. Enjoy your hamburger on a bun with fries and a milkshake. Just make sure that your next meal consists of milk and apple, fruits and/or fresh vegetables and/or salads. A detoxified body can easily deal with a chemically incompatible meal as long as you bolster its alkaline reserve by returning to the A&B Method.

Losing weight is a very stressful process, but whole milk and apples can make it, not only easy, but also healthy. Begin your day with a breakfast of whole milk and apples. You won't be hungry for hours and you'll have a great foundation for the day. Apples stimulate the metabolism and metabolize fat. High in fiber, they help keep blood sugar levels steady for long periods of time that naturally curbs the appetite.

Combined with milk, they are a great way to detoxify your BioChemical Machine on a daily basis.

Finally, it's important to remember that you might experience an initial *healing process*. Don't worry; this will pass after approximately one week. What you would be experiencing is a "shock to the system" as your body begins the hard work of ridding itself of toxins. The good news is that this process is the first step towards getting rid of unwanted pounds.

Chapter 14

BREATHING & EXERCISE:
Key Factors in the Aging Process

Without good health, physical beauty would be impossible. The skin, our largest organ, is not only one of the vital channels for eliminating toxic wastes, but also the most visible evidence of our beauty. Cosmetic industries have developed hundreds of products to pamper the skin, but there are no miracle creams or beauty products that can keep the human body forever young. The body's cells are programmed, biologically, to age and to die. We cannot prevent our body's aging. But it is in our power to decelerate the aging process by 20 to 30 years, by not poisoning ourselves. It is in your power to look and feel, for example, age 50 at age 70.

My mentor, Professor Joachim Seidl, psychology professor at the Academy for Psychoanalysis and Psychotherapy at Munich, once said, "Everybody has three ages.

The numerical, the biological and the psychological." Your age does not have to pigeonhole you—you do not have to feel "old" at 50, 60, 70, or even 90. You can look and feel younger than your numerical age; because you decide what you eat, and what you eat makes a vast difference in the aging process. According to my observation, some individuals are *biologically* 20 to 30 years younger compared to those suffering from a long-standing alkaline deficit. Surely, this must influence the state of our psychological age.

"Nature provides a self-governing mechanism for the maintenance of health," said Dr. Hay.[41] In his research, he was intrigued by the observations of one Col. Robert McCarrison, of the British Army Medical Service, who was posted in the remote Himalayan region of India during the 1800s.

Dr. McCarrison says that the older men of the tribe looked so much like the younger men that he was often not able to tell the one from the other as they worked in the field, or as they swam in the river at the end of the day. They reported living to unbelievable ages; claims which Col. McCarrison, after living among these people for nine years, accepted as genuine. The older men were apparently as efficient as their much younger counterparts, and easily held their own in the strenuous sports of the tribe.[42]

Dr. Hay concluded: "Their life was that of the agrarian, spent outdoors, at active manual labor.

So, oxidation was insured, with little liability of accumulation of the usual unoxidized waste from which we suffer so much in our unwise eating habits."[42]

I made the same observations in Arabia where I met Bedouins who regularly reached their nineties (and beyond). They didn't know arthritis, constipation, allergies, asthma, cancer, arteriosclerosis, diabetes, stroke, or any of our diseases. The oldest living person, actually 135 years of age, was a Bedouin in Lebanon who was videotaped for a story later aired by CNN. His secret, he said, was "sour milk with whole wheat bread every morning." The grandmother of a colleague died in 1994 at 117 years of age. Every morning she ate whole wheat bread and sour milk. Even if she didn't know about the A&B Method, she lived instinctively according to it. Furthermore, she read the newspaper every day and participated actively in society until two years before her death. When she died from the infirmity of her age, she was in excellent shape.

I've dedicated most of *The BioChemical Machine* explaining how the foods you eat can empower your body chemistry. But I don't want to entirely neglect two other factors that play a role in keeping you healthy and looking great: exercise and breathing correctly.

Exercise

A huge problem for our generation is that we are deluged with the wrong information: "Don't eat fat, count calories, and work out, work out, work out!" And people believe it. They buy into the notion that heavy-duty exercise will deliver the results they want.

In our efficiency-driven society, it has been easy for the $32 billion diet industry to make people believe that the more they work on their bodies, the better the results.

So, they join fitness clubs or buy expensive equipment and exercise to the point of exhaustion.

Now, don't get me wrong; physical exertion is an important part of good health. There's no doubt about it. Chronic inactivity leads to devastating consequences. Exercise—*below the point of fatigue*— leads to the important development of your body. But to exercise beyond fatigue leads to deterioration. Everything beyond the fatigue point is damaging because the over-exertion produces acid remains that overload the body.

BioChemical Machine Fact: *Excessive exercise creates acid in the body. You can actually feel it happening—the burning pain in your muscles. That's not because you exercised with heroic endurance; it's because acid attacked your nerve endings.*

That's why athletes have a greater tendency than most to suffer from conditions like arthritis later in life. You should always stop exercising when you feel pain. This is your body signaling to you: enough is enough.

If you haven't exercised for several years, then begin slowly with an easy exercise and give your body the chance to build up its strength, step by step.

- If you hear music you like—then dance.

- Stretching is great. It strengthens the muscles without undue strain.

- Moderate jogging or a brisk walk is fine. Both encourage blood circulation and support your metabolic process.

If you are one of the mislead individuals who went through many fad diets and followed a strenuous daily workout, slow down. You'll find that doing so will make a huge difference in the quality of your life. And if you combine moderate exercise with the A&B Method, you'll get the results you want.

Breathing

Correct breathing has much more impact on our health than generally assumed. Deep breathing exercises massage the abdominal region and, by that action, improve both blood circulation and the lymphatic system. This, in turn, improves the metabolism—thereby, the metabolism of fat.

When we sleep, we breathe far deeper than when we are awake. It is during sleep that we oxidize our waste matter and eliminate much of this through the lungs. Why not replicate the same results when we're awake?

Forced respiration and the perspiration that accompanies exercise expels toxicity from our bodies. The more muscles we use, the more we speed up both respiration and circulation of the blood. Jogging, walking briskly, biking, and swimming are, for this reason, ideal exercises, as all four call into play the larger groups of muscles.

The benefits of exercise are through this massage of the muscles themselves and of the internal organs, through increased respiration, circulation and perspiration. In short, you exhale the toxic waste faster. In combination, moderate exercise and deep breathing are excellent for your BioChemical Machine.

Skin

With the A&B, the skin will regenerate as well, which is not the case with fad diets. I saw people who lost weight with dieting but their skin didn't regenerate at the same time. They had nice, new body shapes but the same old skin. This is not the case with the A&B way. If you give your body the time to regenerate, as well as observe the rules of your body chemistry, your skin will become more elastic. The combination of exercise and the A&B will restore your skin. What is valid for your body muscles is also true for your facial muscles. If, later in life, you choose plastic surgery, it is easier for your doctor to work on healthy skin.

Of course, as you know now, there are many, many wonderful benefits that can be reaped by adapting the A&B Method into your day-to-day life. Losing weight and beautiful skin is just a side effect of ridding your body of years of accumulated poison and returning it to its original, balanced state. Not only will you look and feel great, but also, by balancing your body chemistry you'll boost your immune system and thwart disease. It can even slow down the effects of the aging process.

Following the A&B Method has made a huge difference in the quality of my life.

Now that you know the truth about the closest companion of your existence—your BioChemical Machine—the decision to make a change is yours.

What you do with this knowledge rests solely in your hands.

PART VI

PUTTING THE A&B METHOD TO PRACTICAL USE

CHAPTER 15

GETTING STARTED
A One-Day Suggested Example

While sharing the wonders of the A&B Method with family, friends, and other interested parties over the past seven years, I was often asked, "What is the best way to get started?" I realized that similar to other life challenges, getting started was the toughest part. Therefore, I've included this one-day example to help you along. I am confident that once you begin, the rest of the program will fall quickly into place. Later chapters will provide you with similar quick-start four-week examples for both Level One and Level Two.

BREAKFAST

You can eat either:

A. Milk and apples or other "B"-fruits. Although you might not think this is a complete and healthy breakfast—*it is*. It will satisfy your nutritional requirements and prevent you from becoming hungry over the next three to four hours.

B. Cereal with raisins, bananas and cream (diluted with water), or yogurt/buttermilk

C. Wheat bread topped with one of the following: cottage cheese; cream cheese and honey; bacon and goat's cheese; butter, fresh tomatoes, and salt

D. Bagel with cream cheese

E. Scrambled (whole eggs) with bacon (without bread)

   OR

   scrambled *egg yolks* with smoked bacon *(not fried!),* with bread

There are no limits when you use your imagination to create the perfect BioChemical breakfast.

- Remember the A&B principles: don't eat "A" with "B."

- If you need to drink coffee then use cream (Neutral) instead of milk, ("B") especially if your breakfast includes cereal ("A") or wheat bread ("A").

Remember, coffee is a strong acid-builder. Furthermore, coffee directly affects your heart and circulatory system and interferes with your hormones. Tea affects the brain and central nervous system as well, although much more slowly than coffee. Black tea with its minerals, fluorine, potash, and manganese is a better choice and herbal tea is the best choice.

FROM BREAKFAST TO LUNCH

In the beginning, you might possibly find yourself sometimes hungry in between meals. Don't fret, this is because your body's chemistry is still undergoing changes. The good news is you **can** eat in between meals as long as you choose foods from the Neutral column like mozzarella cheese on tomatoes, a mushroom salad, or any fresh vegetables or lettuce. These can be eaten anytime, 24 hours a day, seven days a week. Salads and vegetables are great. Don't laugh, but even a cooked egg yolk (without the egg white!) with a little bit of mayonnaise is a tasty snack that can be eaten on the A&B Method.

LUNCH

Lunch will likely depend on your particular circumstances. However, some great choices include:

A. All leafy salads including the A&B Power Salad.
B. Mozzarella with tomatoes, basil, vinegar, olive oil, sea salt and pepper.
C. Meat, fried chicken, sausages, or fish with vegetables, salads and "B"-fruits.

Cooked tomatoes or cooked spinach matches perfectly with these meals. Gravies made with cream are also great. Parmesan cheese is fine. It can also be accompanied by unsweetened wine. In order to compensate for the acid-building protein consumption you should try to eat a base-building apple or melon or any "B"-fruit, like peaches, grapefruit, kiwi, or oranges. NO bananas, figs or dates ("A"). Save them for the evening.

FROM AFTERNOON TO DINNER

Vegetables, salads, or any other Neutral-column food can be eaten at any time. However, if you plan to eat pizza, potatoes, rice, noodles or anything else from the "B"-column for dinner, remember the three to four hour waiting period. But if you know that you are going to eat carbohydrates, then you can also eat raisins or bananas or play it safe by choosing Neutrals.

DINNER

Since The A&B Method is not a diet, you can create meals from whatever you like. Your culinary fantasies have no boundaries. Here are just a few examples:

A. A&B Pizza with A&B Sauce.
B. Baked potatoes with olive oil, herbs and cream cheese, and/or butter with herbs and vegetables and/or salad.
C. Fried (natural) rice or (whole wheat) noodles.
D. A&B Power Salad with whole wheat bread, potatoes, rice, noodles and/or any Neutral cheese.
E. Ramses Beans and Ramses Salad or Lentils/ Lentil soup.
F. Smoked ham (Neutral) with wheat bread and salad.
G. A&B-Burger®, or A&B Sandwiches with mayonnaise, tomatoes, lettuce, onions, or Camembert, or salami, or feta and much more.

Beer "A" goes well with all the above.

If you find you're still hungry before bedtime, have an evening snack. Try nuts, raisins, honey, carrots with olive oil, cauliflower with dips (see cookbook in Part IX), or anything else from the Neutral-column. Just keep in mind:

- Whenever you want to switch between "A" and "B" foods, it is best to wait three to four hours.

- Even if you are healthy, remember the BIG SEVEN ESSENTIALS—and the fact that your liver doesn't like working overtime at night.

Chapter 16

FOUR-WEEK EXAMPLE MENU
For Healthy People

LEVEL ONE

Early in 2001, I was approached by the editors of the popular German publication *Petra Magazine*. They indicated that they were familiar with my research and asked if I might be interested in putting the A&B Method to a very public test! Since I was completely confident in the program's simple effectiveness, I immediately jumped at the opportunity. To get them started as quickly as possible, I created a LEVEL ONE, four-week example menu. I have included that very same example in this chapter.

In the June 2001 issue, the editors reported on the A&B experience.

Healthy weight loss! Petra shows you the main points of the new A&B Method. . . .The new A&B Method in Eleonora De Lennart's book is a work of genius, as well as scientifically sound. During her research, De Lennart worked together with physicians, professors, and scientists. . . .It is, says De Lennart, 'about the perfect match of food chemistry and body chemistry.' If one disregards the chemistry, the body is going to be over-acidified, and, as a result, poisoned. The consequences are overweight, loss of energy... Instead, if one provides the body with base-surplus nourishment, not only will the alkaline reserve—a buffer system—build up, healthy chemistry will be restored.

This all sounds scientific and complicated. But in practice this is not the case at all. We [at Petra*] have tried the A&B with success (15.5 lbs. in three weeks) with a little bit of training and a lot of fun. And the great part: one may eat potatoes, spaghetti, pizza and desserts, yet one loses weight nevertheless.*

Don't worry if you can't follow the rules exactly because you have been invited out or you're going to McDonald's. Simply have one or two 'clean' meals. . . Even alcohol is allowed. . . .Frozen fruits and vegetables are fine.

If you want to know more about this Method or want to know more about the delicious A&B menus, read The BioChemical Machine.

Petra Magazine, www.petra.de., June 2001

Furthermore, Mrs. Bigs Moeller, director of the Health and Beauty Department of *Petra*, wrote me a letter on September 2, 2002, confirming, upon my request, her thoughts about the four-week example. She responded:

Dear Eleonora: We recommended in our article [June 1, 2001, No. 6-01] the A&B as basis for a whole nutrition-philosophy and/or as normal four-week program. Kindest regards, Bigs Moeller.

The program designed for and tested by the editors of *Petra* was drawn from the basic principles of the LEVEL ONE chart. Simply put, healthy individuals following the LEVEL ONE chart will successfully rid their BioChemical Machine of the poisons that trigger acid formation. Like the *Petra* editors, you will soon increase your *alkaline reserve*, experience improved health and vitality, and as a bonus side effect, you will correct your weight.

BioChemical Machine Fact: The A&B Method requires that people who have already developed chronic diseases, are obese or are over 40 need to follow the ratio of 80% base-builders and not more than 20% acid-builders as prescribed in LEVEL TWO. This will be outlined in more detail in the following chapter.

So, if your health status follows the requirements for the LEVEL ONE chart and you want to start sampling all the delicious meals you can enjoy while following the A&B Method, read on!

DAY ONE

BREAKFAST:

Milk & Apples

1–2 glasses of whole milk or yogurt with a minimum of 2 large apples (or 3 medium apples), or any kind of "B"-fruits from the Neutral or "B"-column (bananas, figs, and dates are "A"). Apples are high in fiber. A medium apple contains 9 to 10 grams of fiber, a good portion of the 20 to 35 grams you need every day. One glass of milk (250 ml) contains 8 grams fat, a fragment of the 60 to 80 grams fat that are healthy for a moderately active person. By drinking whole milk (moderate base-builder) and eating apples (strong base-builders) you will build a strong alkaline foundation for *the day*.

OPTIONAL:

Bagel with cream cheese
    OR
Wheat bread topped with cottage cheese
Cream cheese and honey
Bacon and goat's cheese
Butter, fresh tomatoes and salt
    OR
Scrambled (whole eggs)
    with either:
Smoked bacon (without bread), OR scrambled egg yolks with smoked bacon (not fried!), with bread;
    OR

Classic Cereal Breakfast
Large bowl of cereal (whole grain, without sugar), <u>with either:</u>
Yogurt or sour cream
    OR
Cream (diluted with filtered water). May be served with bananas, blueberries, and/or raisins or dates, dried figs, honey, and/or all kinds of Neutral nuts, including peanuts from the "A" column.
    OR
Whole grain toast with butter and honey, or with butter or mayonnaise and/or any Neutral cheese above 60% fat, (such as cream cheese, cottage cheese, Camembert, goat's milk cheese), topped with chives, tomatoes, onions or any other vegetable and herb; or any Neutral meat/sausage, such as smoked or rolled ham.

- Drink tea, herbal tea, water or coffee. Instead of milk, *put cream diluted with water* in your coffee if you eat bread, cereal, or bagel.
- But you can drink your coffee with regular milk if you eat eggs. However, the base-building cream *makes good for the acid-building* coffee.

WHAT ABOUT *SNACKS*?

If you want to have something between meals, you may eat Neutrals 24 hours a day, 7 days a week. Try mozzarella cheese on tomatoes, mushroom salad, or any fresh vegetables, lettuce, or salads. Also, a couple stalks of raw cauliflower dipped in chunky blue cheese dressing, fresh and made without preservatives, not only tastes good but also work wonders.

And, of course, fruits! Neutral or "B"-cheese with "B" or Neutral fruits taste delicious. Keep in mind that some fruits belong to "B," others to "A," but blueberries are Neutral.

LUNCH:

There is no limit to the number of vegetables, salads, sprouts, and herbs you can have at lunch. You don't need to add ALL of the following suggested vegetables to you're A&B Power Salad, but it would be great if you did. By eating so many different vegetables and salads, your metabolism has it all.

A&B POWER SALAD*

Lettuce (romaine, iceberg, limestone, red leaf, watercress, or any other lettuce, broken into bite-size pieces)
Tomatoes, sliced or diced into cubes
Cucumber, sliced or diced into cubes
Carrots, chopped or sliced
Cauliflower, chopped
Broccoli, chopped
White and/or red cabbage, chopped
Sprouts/soy sprouts
Spinach, chopped
Onions, sliced or diced into cubes
Scallions, sliced
Parsley, chopped
Chive, chopped
Oil to taste (olive, flaxseed, sesame, etc.)
Apple vinegar (opt: balsamic) or fresh lemon juice to taste
Salt (sea salt, herb salt, Bio-salt) to taste
Pepper to taste

1. Cut up vegetables. In a large bowl, combine all vegetables.

2. In a small bowl, combine oil, vinegar, salt, pepper, and chives (or OPTIONAL salad dressings, such as chunky blue cheese dressing or mayonnaise dip. See cookbook in Part IX). Pour over salad.

*If you are a working person and bring your food from home, then eat either fruits (from the "B"-group) or any kind of salads, according to the A&B Power Salad.

You can eat your salads and fruits with cottage cheese, goat or ewe's milk cheese, feta, mozzarella, cream cheese, Roquefort, ricotta, Camembert, or anything from the Neutral group. You will realize that you can buy almost the same foods at salad bars in supermarkets, delis, and restaurants.

• The A&B Power Salad can be eaten with Neutral cheese (cottage, ricotta, Camembert, cream Brie, etc.) or "B"-cheese (Cheddar, Colby, Gouda, etc.), Neutral meat (salami, smoked or cured ham, dried meat, etc.) or "B"-meat (cooked meat, cooked sausages, etc.), Neutral fish (smoked, marinated, or raw fish), or "B"-fish (cooked fish). If you eat the A&B Power Salad with "B" or Neutral meat, "B" or Neutral fish, or "B" or Neutral cheese, you should eat it with "B"-fruits and, of course, with anything from the Neutral column.

• The A&B Power Salad can also be eaten with "A"-foods, such as (steamed) potatoes, rice, pasta, and, of course, all kinds of whole grain breads, such as whole wheat, rye, potato, Canadian oat, etc. (see cookbook, A&B Sandwiches). But remember Essential #5, the biological liver rhythm. Your liver doesn't like "A"-food before late afternoon/early evening. If you choose to eat the A&B Power Salad with wheat bread, potatoes, rice, or pasta, you may also eat bananas, grapes, figs, dates, nuts, raisins, honey, and, of course, anything from the Neutral group. In this case you can choose any "A" or Neutral DESSERT from the cookbook.

HELPFUL TIP: *Most people quickly tire of cutting up vegetables day in and day out. In order to have this vital food available any time you are hungry, you should prepare a huge bowl of raw vegetables sufficient for a couple of days. Vegetables don't perish quickly and can be kept refrigerated for several days. Chop or slice carrots and white and/or red cabbage and prepare cauliflower and broccoli according to your taste. Put chopped onions in a separate bowl that can be closed, so that your refrigerator will not smell. Prepare (wash and cut) only a limited amount of fresh leafy greens/lettuce, since they perish very quickly. When you come home, you just need to take a bit from every bowl and mix with oil, vinegar, and sea salt.*

Snacks from Lunch to Dinner:

If you ate your lunch with Neutrals, you have no restrictions. If you ate your lunch with cooked meat, cooked sausages, or cooked fish ("B"-group foods), you may continue with (base-building) "B"-fruits. But don't forget the waiting period of three to four hours in regard to the pizza ("A"-group) you might eat for dinner. If you ate your lunch with potatoes, bread, rice, or pasta, you may continue to eat fruits from the "A"-group or anything from the Neutral group with emphasis on base-builders.

DINNER:

Pizza A&B Four Seasons
2 cups whole wheat flour
1 tablespoon yeast
1 1/2 cups water
1 tablespoon salt
1 cup Ricotta cheese
1/2 cup heavy cream
3 cloves garlic
1 teaspoon dried parsley
1 teaspoon basil
1 teaspoon oregano
2 cups mozzarella, shredded
2 tablespoons olive oil
1 tablespoon butter
1 tablespoon olive oil
Broccoli, small pieces (quantity to taste)
Cauliflower, quantity to taste
Mushrooms, quantity to taste, sliced
1/2 eggplant, sliced 3/4 inch
1 large onion, sliced into rings
Olives, quantity to taste

A&B Pizza Sauce: In a food processor, combine Ricotta cheese, garlic, cream, oregano, parsley, dried basil. Process until a paste forms. Slowly add oil; set aside.
A&B Pizza Dough: In a medium mixing bowl combine flour, yeast, oil, salt, and water. Stir mixture; knead with your hands till dough is firm but moist (if necessary, add more water, 1 tablespoon at a time). Let dough rest for 1 hour.

1. Knead dough again with your hands. Cover and let rise for 20 minutes in a warm place.
2. Preheat oven to 350°F. Sprinkle whole wheat flour over greased baking sheet. Roll out dough and place on baking sheet.
3. Spread pizza sauce evenly over dough. Top with broccoli, cauliflower, mushrooms, eggplant, onions, and olives. Sprinkle mozzarella evenly over pizza. Place baking sheet on lowest shelf in oven (or the floor of a gas oven) and bake until crust is firm and golden brown, 15 to 20 minutes. Serve warm.

149

Other Dinner Options:

Ramses Salad
With Whole Wheat Bread or Whole Wheat Pita Bread
5–6 fresh hot peppers, such as jalapeno
2–3 large tomatoes
1 head of lettuce
6 large cloves of garlic
2 large onions
1 tablespoon coriander
1 bunch cilantro
1 tablespoon cumin
Salt and pepper to taste
1/2 cup vinegar and
1/2 cup olive oil

In a food processor, combine pepper, tomatoes, onions, lettuce, garlic, salt, pepper, vinegar, oil, and herbs. Process until well blended to form a pulp. *TIP: Put the remaining Ramses Salad in a jar. Cover with olive oil, 2-inches above pulp. Refrigerate for later use.*

A&B-BURGER® or A&B SANDWICH
(See cookbook). Or try whole wheat bread with butter, mayonnaise, bacon, and/or cheese above 60% fat (cream cheese, Camembert, Brie, cottage cheese, or any other Neutral cheese) with raw vegetables and dill spears

DESSERT:

You can choose any "A" or Neutral dessert from the cookbook, such as:

Banana Cream
2 pound bananas
2 cups heavy cream, whipped
1/2 teaspoon vanilla
1/4 cup almonds, minced
Raisins
Honey to taste

In a processor, combine bananas with whipped cream, 1/2 teaspoon vanilla, and honey. Process until mixture is firm. Garnish with raisins; refrigerate.

Snacks From Dinner To Bedtime:
Choose anything from the Neutral group with an emphasis on base-building nuts, honey, vegetables, salads and "A"-fruits.

DAY TWO

BREAKFAST:
Same as Day One

LUNCH:

Broccoli Milanese*   2 servings
4 stalks broccoli, washed and stems cut off
2 tablespoons butter
2 teaspoons fresh lemon juice
Seasoning to taste

1. Cut each broccoli stem into individual florets. Place in vegetable steamer over boiling water until tender, covered, for 7 minutes.
2. In a small saucepan, melt butter. Combine with lemon juice. Pour sauce over hot broccoli. Season to taste.

COMPATIBLE with "A," "B," and Neutral Groups

*Optional for Working People: Same as Day One

151

DINNER:

New Potatoes Marseilles   *2 servings*

5 small red-skinned potatoes, unpeeled
(Alternative: 1–2 New Jersey potatoes, russet potatoes or other type)
2–3 tablespoons butter, melted
1/4 cup fresh parsley, chopped
Salt and pepper to taste

1. In a vegetable steamer, bring water to a boil. Place washed, potatoes over boiling water for 20 minutes. Cook until tender. Remove from heat. Place potatoes in a large bowl. Let stand until potatoes are cool enough to handle.
2. Cut unpeeled potatoes into quarter-inch slices. Place on baking sheet and sprinkle evenly with butter. Sprinkle with seasoning and place as close as possible to heat of broiler until crusty and golden, approximately 10 minutes.

COMPATIBLE with "A" and Neutral

Other Dinner Options:

RAMSES SALAD
Or
A&B SANDWICH,

1–2 slices wheat bread with fresh butter, bacon, and/or cheese above 60% fat (cream cheese, Camembert, Brie, cottage cheese, etc.) with raw vegetables and/or mixed salads.

COMPATIBLE with "A" and Neutral

DESSERT: "A" and/or Neutral

Snacks From Dinner To Bedtime:
Choose anything from Neutral, or continue with "A"-fruits and/or nuts and raisins.

DAY THREE

BREAKFAST:
Same as Day One

LUNCH:

Chicken Thighs with Vegetables*   4 servings
8 pieces chicken
1/4 cup grated Parmesan cheese
2 tablespoons butter
4 tablespoons butter, melted
1 cup grated carrots
1 cup broccoli, chopped
1 onion, chopped
Salt to taste
Pepper to taste
Oregano to taste

1. Preheat oven to 350°F. Place chicken in a baking sheet. Sprinkle the chicken with butter and Parmesan cheese. Bake until chicken is tender, for 45 minutes.
2. In a frying pan, melt butter over medium-high heat. Add carrots, broccoli, and onion and cook, tossing often, for 5 minutes, until broccoli is crisp-tender.
3. Serve chicken mixed in with vegetables.

COMPATIBLE with "B" and Neutral

*Optional for Working People: Same as Day One or Fried Chicken.

DINNER:

Pasta Parisian   4 servings

1/2 pound rigatoni (or other pasta)
1 large eggplant
1 cup ricotta cheese or cottage cheese
1/2 cup heavy cream, diluted with water
1/2 cup olive oil
2 large cloves garlic, crushed through a press
2 carrots, cut into thin strips, about 3 inches long
2 celery stalks, cut into thin strips, about 3 inches long
4 onions, finely chopped
Soy sauce to taste
1 teaspoon oregano
1 teaspoon basil
Cayenne pepper to taste

1. Cut eggplant into 3/4-inch cubes. Put eggplant in a strainer. Sprinkle sufficient salt over eggplant. Let stand until fluid drains off, 45 minutes.
2. In a saucepan, cook pasta in boiling salted water until tender but firm. Remove from heat and drain.
3. In a deep frying pan (a wok is preferred), cook onions and garlic in hot oil until brown. Add 3/4-inch eggplant. Season with soy sauce, oregano, basil, and cayenne pepper. Reduce heat, cook, stirring occasionally, at least 1/2 hour. Add ricotta or cottage cheese and 1/2 cup heavy cream. Add mixture to rigatoni. Mix well.

COMPATIBLE with "A" and Neutral

OPTIONAL: Same as Day One

DAY FOUR

BREAKFAST:
Same as Day One

LUNCH:

Cauliflower Soufflé Côte d'Azur*   4 servings
1 large cauliflower, cored and broken into small florets
3 tablespoons oil
2 egg yolks
1/4 cup parsley, chopped
1 pinch sweet Hungarian or other paprika
1 pinch nutmeg

1. Preheat oven to 350°F.
2. In a saucepan, cook cauliflower in boiling salted water until just tender, about 10 minutes. Remove from heat.
3. In a small soufflé dish, heat oil.
4. Whisk two egg yolks with 3 tablespoons oil, nutmeg, pepper, and parsley.
5. Spread mixture over cauliflower. Bake until soufflé is golden brown, about 10–15 minutes.

Note: Cauliflower contains pantothenic acid which detoxifies cells and plays a vital role in the biochemical reactions within the body—and it creates new skin.

COMPATIBLE with "A", "B", and Neutral

*Optional for Working People: Same as Day One

155

DINNER:

A&B Power Salad
(Same as Day One)
OPTIONAL: Potatoes may be added to the A&B Power Salad

1. In a vegetable steamer, place unpeeled potatoes over boiling water for 20 minutes.
2. Cook until tender.
3. Remove from heat. Place tomatoes in a large bowl. Let stand until potatoes are cool enough to handle. Peel potatoes.
4. Cut potatoes into 1/4-inch slices or dice into small cubes. Add potatoes, mayonnaise, or dip/dressing to the A&B Power Salad. Mix well.

Compatible with anything from the Neutral group, "A", or "B"

Optional: Same as Day One

DAY FIVE

BREAKFAST:
Same as Day One

LUNCH:

Cabbage Budapest*   2–3 servings
1 white cabbage, sliced
1 pound onions, diced
2 cups vegetable broth (or bouillon cubes)
2 cups heavy cream
2 tablespoons butter
1 cup sour cream
Sea salt to taste
2 teaspoons Hungarian or other paprika
Soy sauce to taste

1. In a large saucepan, sauté onions in butter until golden brown. Add vegetable broth or bouillon cubes and sea salt.
2. Place cabbage in saucepan and cook for 15 20 minutes. Remove from heat and drain cabbage.
3. Combine heavy cream with paprika and season to taste. Sprinkle mixture over cabbage. Let stand 10 minutes.

COMPATIBLE with "A", "B", and Neutral

*Optional for Working People: Same as Day One

DINNER:

Roast Chicken Hawaii   4 servings

1 whole chicken, about 3 pounds
2 tablespoons butter
2 tablespoons olive oil
Pineapples, diced
1 teaspoon dried thyme
Salt and pepper to taste
1 cup dry white wine

1. Preheat oven to 350°F. Season chicken inside and out with salt and pepper. Place 1/2 teaspoon thyme in cavity. Tie legs together and rub butter over skin. Place in a large roasting pan.
2. Roast chicken for 15 minutes. Arrange diced pineapples around chicken. Sprinkle remaining thyme over chicken. Pour dry white wine over all and bake 1 hour and 15 minutes. Add water (or cream) when wine evaporates, approximately 5 minutes.

COMPATIBLE with "B" and Neutral

OPTIONAL: Same as Day One

DAY SIX

BREAKFAST:
Same as Day One

LUNCH:

Waldorf Astoria Salad*

2 cups diced apples (about 2 medium apples)
2 sweet oranges, diced (without seeds)
1/2 pound cooked chicken, diced (good use of leftovers)
1 cup celery, coarsely chopped
1 cup mayonnaise
1 cup sour cream
4 tablespoons heavy cream, whipped
1/2 cup coarsely chopped walnuts
1 dash cognac
2 tablespoons lemon juice or vinegar
1 dash salt

In a medium bowl, combine all ingredients, except whipped cream, sour cream, and walnuts. Mix well. Chill thoroughly. Add whipped cream, sour cream, and walnuts before serving. Serve on lettuce. Leftovers should be refrigerated.

COMPATIBLE with "B" and Neutral

*Optional for Working People: Same as Day One

DINNER:

A&B Power Salad
(Same as Day One)

OPTIONAL: Same as Day One

DAY SEVEN

BREAKFAST:
Same as Day One

LUNCH:

Mozzarella with Tomatoes *   2 servings
2 large tomatoes, sliced
1 ball of mozzarella, sliced
Fresh basil
Vinegar
Olive oil
Salt
Pepper

1. Cut tomatoes and mozzarella in thin slices. Arrange on a plate.
2. In a small bowl, combine vinegar and oil. Pour mixture over mozzarella and tomatoes. Add salt and pepper to taste. Garnish with fresh basil.

COMPATIBLE with "A", "B", and Neutral

*Optional for Working People: Same as Day One

DINNER:

Eggplant Normandy   4 servings

2 large eggplants (or 4 small)
6 cloves garlic, crushed through a press
4 small onions, peeled
2 medium tomatoes, pureed
2 cups olive oil
1 bunch parsley, chopped
1 bunch cilantro, chopped
Salt
Pepper
Celery salt

1. Preheat oven to 300°F.
2. With a sharp knife, remove stem head of eggplants. Cut eggplants into 1/2-inch slices.
3. Chop cilantro and parsley. Puree tomatoes. Add garlic. Mix well.
4. In a large saucepan, heat cooking oil. Place eggplants in oil. Fry until brown.
5. On a baking sheet, place eggplant slices. Sprinkle tomato-cilantro-parsley mixture over eggplants. Bake for 20 minutes, until crispy. Season to taste.

COMPATIBLE with "B" and Neutral (if eaten without tomatoes, also compatible with "A")

OPTIONAL: Same as Day One

DAY EIGHT

BREAKFAST:
Same as Day One

LUNCH:

Meatballs *   4 servings
2 pounds ground meat
2 onions, chopped
2 onions, sliced
2 stalks celery, chopped
3–4 cloves garlic
1/2 bunch parsley
1 large can Italian peeled tomatoes, 12 ounces
Butter to taste
Soy sauce to taste
Salt to taste
Pepper to taste
Celery salt, oregano, basil to taste

1. In a food processor or blender combine chopped onions, celery, garlic, parsley, salt, pepper, celery salt, oregano and basil. Process vegetables. Add meat and spices. Process until a puree forms. Form meatballs, 1 1/2-inch diameter.
2. In a frying pan, combine butter and sliced onions until lightly brown. Add salt, pepper, oregano, parsley, celery salt, and basil. Mix well. Add Italian peeled tomatoes. Chop up while cooking. Add meatballs and cook (low), turning, about 1 hour. Add soy sauce to taste.

COMPATIBLE with "B" and Neutral

*Optional for Working People: Same as Day One

DINNER:

Creamy Cauliflower Soup   4 servings

6 cups (distilled) water
2 medium cauliflowers, cored and coarsely chopped
1 onion, chopped
1 clove garlic, crushed through a press
2 tablespoons butter
1 tablespoon olive oil
2 stalks celery, chopped
8 scallions, chopped
2 tablespoons vegetable broth (or bouillon cubes)
1/8 teaspoon fresh ground black pepper
1/8 teaspoon nutmeg
1 teaspoon dried basil
1/2 teaspoon dried thyme
1 teaspoon dried marjoram
1/2 teaspoon celery or sea salt

In a large saucepan, melt butter and heat oil. Add scallions, onions, garlic, cauliflower and celery. Season with salt and pepper to taste. Cook over medium heat for several minutes, stirring frequently. Add vegetable broth or the water and bouillon; bring to a boil. Add basil, thyme, marjoram. Simmer, covered, over medium heat until cauliflower is tender, for 10–15 minutes. Remove cover and cool slightly. In blender, process until soup is smooth and creamy. Add nutmeg to taste.

COMPATIBLE with "A", "B", and Neutral

OPTIONAL: Same as Day One

DAY NINE

BREAKFAST:
Same as Day One

LUNCH:

Mushrooms Lyon*   2–3 servings
1/2 pound mushrooms
2 tablespoons butter
1 tablespoon fresh lemon juice
Dash sea salt
Dash garlic salt
Soy sauce

1   Wash mushrooms; cut and discard ends from stems. Cut mushrooms into slices.
2   In a saucepan, melt butter. Add mushrooms, tossing lightly in butter, until soft. Add lemon juice. Season to taste.

COMPATIBLE with "A", "B", and Neutral

*Optional for Working People: Same as Day One

DINNER:

Spaghetti à la Toscana   4 servings
1/2 pound spaghetti
4 onions, chopped
2 large cloves garlic, crushed through a press
1 1/2 pounds mushrooms, sliced
2 tablespoons butter
1/2 pound grated fresh cheese (above 60% fat)
1 cup heavy cream

1 teaspoon fresh basil, chopped
1 pinch salt
1 pinch pepper
1 teaspoon basil
1 teaspoon oregano

1. In a medium saucepan, cook onions and mushrooms in butter until softened but not brown. Add garlic, salt, and pepper to taste. Add fresh cheese. Cook until melted. Add cream. Mix well; set aside.
2. In a large saucepan, cook pasta in boiling salted water until tender but firm. Remove from heat and drain. Sprinkle mixture over spaghetti. Sprinkle fresh basil and oregano to taste.

COMPATIBLE with "A" and Neutral

OPTIONAL: Same as Day One

DAY TEN

BREAKFAST:
Same as Day One

LUNCH:

Zurich "Geschnetzeltes"*   4 servings
1 1/2 pounds beef or veal
1 pound mushrooms, sliced
1 can green peas
1 cup heavy cream
2 large onions, chopped
4 cloves garlic, crushed through a press
Celery salt to taste
Garlic powder to taste
Salt and pepper to taste

1. Cut meat in 1/2-inch slices. Season with celery salt and pepper.

2. In a small frying pan, combine butter, onions, and garlic. Heat until lightly brown. Add meat and cook, turning, until brown. Reduce heat and add mushrooms, seasoning, and heavy cream. Cook, stirring occasionally, about 1 hour. Add peas and season to taste.

COMPATIBLE with "B" and Neutral

*Optional for Working People: Same as Day One

DINNER:

Potato Salad d'Alsace   4 servings
6 new potatoes, unpeeled
Beef salami, diced into cubes (optional: smoked fish), quantity to taste
1 fresh cucumber, sliced
1 large tomato, cut into small cubes
2 large pickles (sour or sweet dill), chopped into very thin slices
1/2 bunch chives, chopped
Scallions, to taste, chopped
1 onion, chopped
Mayonnaise and/or chunky Blue Cheese dressing, to taste
Olive or any other natural oil to taste
Vinegar to taste
Salt, pepper, and celery salt to taste

1. In a vegetable steamer, place potatoes over boiling water for 20 to 30 minutes. Cook until tender. Remove from heat. Place potatoes in a large bowl. Let stand until potatoes are cool enough to handle. Peel potatoes. Cut potatoes into 1/2-inch cubes.
2. Add oil, vinegar, vegetables, cucumber, salami (or fish), and mayonnaise to potatoes. Mix well.

COMPATIBLE with "A" and Neutral

OPTIONAL: Same as Day One

DAY ELEVEN

BREAKFAST:
Same as Day One

LUNCH:

<u>A&B Power Salad*</u>
(Same as Day One)

Compatible with anything from the Neutral group, "A", or "B"

*Optional for Working People: Same as Day One

DINNER:

DON'T FORGET TO PREPARE YOUR DINNER AHEAD OF TIME:
Soaking of the beans requires 3 to 4 hours and cooking time of 4 to 5 hours!

<u>Ramses Beans & Ramses Salad</u>
*Old Egyptian recipe; beans should be eaten with Ramses Salad to ensure proper digestion. **(Optional:** add onions, dressed with vinegar, pepper, salt, and cumin. Crush onions with your hand to enhance the flavor.)*

2 pounds small fava beans
1 pound skinless fava beans
1 pound Garbanzo beans (chickpeas)
1/2 pound yellow lentils
1 large bulb of garlic, crushed through a press
2 tablespoons cumin
2 tablespoons dried coriander
Salt to taste
Pepper to taste

1. Wash beans and lentils separately. In a big bowl, put fava beans, skinless fava beans, and Garbanzo beans. Cover beans with plenty of (distilled) cold water. Soak beans for 3–4 hours. Remove from water.
2. In a large saucepan, bring water to a boil. Add fava beans and Garbanzo beans. Cover with water, 4 inches above. Reduce heat.
3. Check the water level every hour, adding water if necessary.
4. Simmer over medium-low heat for 4–5 hours, until soft. As soon as beans are soft, add lentils. Let cook, for 1 hour, until soft. Add garlic, cumin, coriander, salt, and pepper. Let stand for 30 minutes. Serve warm. Top the Ramses Beans with Ramses Salad (OPTIONAL: mash beans with mixer and top it with Ramses Salad).

COMPATIBLE with "A", "B", and Neutral

HELPFUL TIP: *Leftovers can be stored in freezer. Put small portions in bowls or plastic bags for later.*

Ramses Salad

5–6 fresh hot peppers, such as jalapenos
2–3 large tomatoes
1 head of lettuce
6 large cloves of garlic
2 large onions
1 tablespoon coriander
1 bunch cilantro
1 tablespoon cumin
Salt and pepper to taste
1/2 cup vinegar
1/2 cup olive oil

In a food processor, combine all ingredients. Process until well blended to form a pulp. Top Ramses Beans with 3 tablespoons Ramses Salad.

HELPFUL TIP: *In a jar, put remaining Ramses Salad. Cover with olive oil, 2-inches above pulp. Refrigerate for later use (for example, with whole wheat bread or pita).*

DAY TWELVE

BREAKFAST:
Same as Day One

LUNCH:

Fettuccine Alfredo*   4–6 servings
1 pound fettuccine
8 tablespoons butter, softened
1/4 cup heavy cream
1 cup grated mozzarella cheese
Freshly ground pepper

1. Cook pasta in boiling salted water until tender but firm. Remove from heat and drain.
2. Place fettuccine in a warm bowl or on a serving platter. Add butter, cream, and half the mozzarella cheese. Toss fettuccine noodles gently until they are evenly coated. Serve immediately, topped with pepper and remaining mozzarella cheese.

COMPATIBLE with "A" and Neutral

*Optional for Working People: Same as Day One

DINNER:

Baked Sole with Oranges   4 servings

1 1/2 pounds sole fillets
1/2 teaspoon salt
1/4 teaspoon pepper
1 teaspoon soy flour
1/4 cup fresh orange juice
1/4 cup fresh lemon juice
1 whole orange

1. Preheat oven to 425°F.
2. Arrange fish in a baking dish large enough to hold fillets flat in a single layer. Season with salt and pepper. Add orange juice and lemon juice. Cover and refrigerate 1 hour.
3. Use a serrated knife to cut away peel from orange. Cut between membranes to remove whole sections. Place in a small bowl and set aside.
4. Remove fish from refrigerator and cover dish tightly with aluminum foil. Bake 8–10 minutes, until firm and opaque throughout.
5. Transfer fillets to serving plate. Pour cooking liquid into a small saucepan. Dissolve soy flour in 2 tablespoons cold water. Stir into liquid in saucepan and bring to a boil over medium-high heat, stirring until thickened, for 1 minute. Spread sauce over fillets; garnish with orange slices.

COMPATIBLE with "B" and Neutral

OPTIONAL: Same as Day One

DAY THIRTEEN

BREAKFAST:
Same as Day One

LUNCH:

Chef Salad*
Lettuce (quantity to taste)
Tomatoes, sliced or diced into cubes
Cucumbers, thinly sliced
Broccoli, sliced
Cauliflower, sliced
Carrots, thinly sliced
Onions, sliced or diced into cubes
1–2 boiled eggs, sliced
Swiss cheese, thinly sliced
Smoked ham, sliced
Cooked turkey or chicken, rectangular slices
Oil to taste
Vinegar to taste
Salt to taste
Pepper to taste
Mayonnaise (OPTIONAL: dip or salad dressing)

Cut vegetables. In a large bowl, combine all vegetables, smoked and/or cooked ham, cooked turkey, or chicken. Add oil, vinegar, salt, and pepper. Add mayonnaise, dip, or dressing.

COMPATIBLE with "B" and Neutral

*Optional for Working People: Same as Day One

DINNER:

Mozzarella Pizza
A&B Pizza Dough and A&B Pizza Sauce
(Same as Day One; also see cookbook)
3 cups mozzarella cheese (about 12 ounces), shredded
2 tablespoons pine nuts

1. Prepare pizza dough.
2. Prepare pizza sauce.
3. Preheat oven to 350°F.
4. Spread pizza sauce evenly over dough. Top with mozzarella and pine nuts. Place baking sheet on lowest shelf in oven (or the floor of a gas oven). Bake until crust is firm and golden brown, 15 to 20 minutes. Serve warm.

COMPATIBLE with "A" and Neutral

OPTIONAL: Same as Day One

DAY FOURTEEN

BREAKFAST:
Same as Day One

LUNCH:

Cabbage Budapest*   4 servings
1 white cabbage, sliced
1 pound onions, diced
2 cups vegetable water (or bouillon cube)
2 cups heavy cream
1 cup sour cream
2 tablespoons butter
Sea salt to taste
2 teaspoons Hungarian paprika
Soy sauce to taste

1. In a large saucepan, cook onions in butter until golden brown. Add vegetable broth and sea salt to taste.
2. Place cabbage in saucepan and cook for 15–20 minutes. Remove from heat and drain.
3. Combine heavy cream and sour cream with paprika and season to taste. Sprinkle mixture over cabbage. Let stand 10 minutes.

COMPATIBLE with "A", "B", and Neutral

*Optional for Working People: Same as Day One

DINNER:

Austrian Baked Potatoes "Arnold"   4 servings

Potatoes, unpeeled, quantity to taste
Butter, 1 tablespoon for each potato
Sour cream or ready-to-buy fresh creamy Italian garlic dip or fresh sour
cream dip without preservatives
Herbs, parsley, and chives
Salt
Pepper
Aluminum wrap

1.   With a sharp knife, make a lengthwise cut across each potato.
     Season potatoes with salt and pepper to taste. Top each potato
     with a tablespoon of butter. Wrap each potato in aluminum
     wrap.
2.   Preheat oven to 400°F. Place potatoes on baking sheet. Bake
     until tender, about 45 minutes.
3.   In a bowl, mix sour cream with parsley and chives to taste.
4.   Serve warm (in aluminum wrap).

COMPATIBLE with "A" and Neutral

OPTIONAL: Same as Day One

DAY FIFTEEN

BREAKFAST:
Same as Day One

LUNCH:

Mozzarella with Tomatoes*   2 servings
2 large tomatoes, sliced
1 ball mozzarella, sliced
Fresh basil
Vinegar to taste
Olive oil to taste
Salt to taste
Pepper to taste

1. Cut tomatoes and mozzarella in thin slices. Arrange on a plate.
2. In a small bowl, combine vinegar and oil. Pour mixture over mozzarella and tomatoes. Add salt and pepper to taste. Garnish with fresh basil.

COMPATIBLE with "A", "B", and Neutral

*Optional for Working People: Same as Day One

DINNER:

Italian Stuffed Green Peppers   4 servings

(Optional: tomato or zucchini)
2 pounds ground meat
2 middle-size onions, sliced
2 middle-size onions, cut in halves
8 green peppers (or 8 zucchini or 8 large tomatoes)
5 cloves garlic, crushed through a press (or garlic powder to taste)
1/2 bunch parsley, chopped
1/2 bunch cilantro, chopped
1/2 bunch dill, chopped
2 tablespoons butter or olive oil
1 bouillon cube
Pinch saffron
Juice of 1 lemon

1. In a food processor or blender, combine parsley, cilantro, garlic, and dill. Process until a puree forms.
2. In a large bowl, combine meat, eggs, vegetable puree, and seasonings (except saffron and lemon). Blend well.
3. With a sharp knife, cut off tops of green peppers (or tomatoes or zucchini). Carefully remove seeds and veins, leaving stems intact.
4. Stuff vegetable with mixture.
5. Preheat oven to 350°F. In a large baking dish, melt 2 tablespoons of butter (or oil), bake 2 onions, cut in halves until softened. Arrange vegetables.
6. In a small frying pan, heat 1 cup of water and add 1 bouillon cube, saffron and lemon juice. Add to vegetables. Bake until vegetables have absorbed most of the juice. Remove from oven. Add sour cream. Let stand, 20 minutes. Serve warm.

COMPATIBLE with "B" and Neutral

OPTIONAL: Same as Day One

DAY SIXTEEN

BREAKFAST:
Same as Day One

LUNCH:

Sylvia's Tuna Salad*   4 servings
1 (6 1/2 ounce) can tuna, in oil or water
1/4 cup capers, cut in halves
3 tablespoons chopped onions
2 tablespoons mustard
1/2 cup pickles, diced
1/3 cup parsley, chopped
Olive oil, quantity to taste
1 teaspoon fresh lemon juice (or vinegar)
1/4 teaspoon pepper
Salt to taste
Garlic salt to taste

In a medium bowl, mash tuna with oil and mustard. Add onions, lemon juice, pickles, capers, salt, and pepper. Mix well. Serve on lettuce. Garnish with remaining capers or pickle slices.

COMPATIBLE with "B" and Neutral

*Optional for Working People: Same as Day One

DINNER:

A&B Power Salad
(Same as Day One with anything from the Neutral group, A, or B)

OPTIONAL: Same as Day One

DAY SEVENTEEN

BREAKFAST:
Same as Day One

LUNCH:

Macaroni & Cheese*   4 servings
1/2 pound macaroni
3 cup shredded mozzarella
4–5 cloves garlic, crushed through a press
1 teaspoon oregano
1 teaspoon thyme

1. In a large saucepan, cook macaroni in boiling salted water until tender but firm. Remove from heat and drain.
2. Combine mozzarella with oregano, thyme, and garlic. Sprinkle mixture over macaroni.
3. Preheat oven to 300°F. Place macaroni in a greased baking dish. Bake until macaroni is golden brown and crisp, 20 minutes.

COMPATIBLE with "A" and Neutral

*Optional for Working People: Same as Day One

DINNER:

Crispy Rice Balls St. Tropez   4 servings

1 cup brown rice
1 1/2 tablespoons butter
4 cups chicken broth or bouillon
Wheat or soy flour
3 egg yolks
1/4 pound mozzarella cheese, cut into 20 cubes
1/4 cup grated cheese (above 60% fat)
1/4 teaspoon freshly ground pepper
1/4 teaspoon grated nutmeg
1 tablespoon parsley, minced
Bread crumbs

1. In a medium saucepan, melt butter over medium-low heat. Add rice and cook, stirring, 2–3 minutes. Add 2 cups of broth (or bouillon cubes). Cook rice, stirring 5–6 minutes. Add 1 more cup broth. Cook until fluid is almost absorbed, 4–5 minutes. Gradually add remaining broth. Cook, continuously stirring, until rice is tender but firm, about 10–15 minutes. Remove from heat. Let cool.
2. In a large bowl, beat 1 egg yolk. Add rice along with cheese, parsley, pepper, and nutmeg. Blend well. Cover mixture and refrigerate at least 1 hour, until chilled.
3. After 1 hour, in a small bowl, beat 2 egg yolks with 2 teaspoons water; set aside.
4. Scoop mixture. Place mozzarella in center. Shape rice with the palms of your hands into balls (1 1/2 inches). Roll balls in flour. Roll balls in egg yolks. Coat balls with bread crumbs. Place rice balls on a baking sheet. Cover with plastic wrap. Refrigerate for 2 hours.
5. In a heavy saucepan, heat 3 inches of oil to 375°F; then add rice balls. Fry, occasionally turning, for 3–5 minutes, until golden brown. Remove with a slotted spoon. Drain on paper towels. Serve at once.

COMPATIBLE with "A" and Neutral

OPTIONAL: Same as Day One

DAY EIGHTEEN

BREAKFAST:
Same as Day One

LUNCH:

Smoked Salmon and Parmesan*   4 servings
3 ounces thinly sliced smoked salmon
1/4 teaspoon hot pepper sauce
Dash of lemon juice
8 ounces natural cream cheese, softened
1 cup fresh dill or parsley
3/4 cup grated Parmesan cheese (about 3 ounces)

1. Preheat oven to 400°F. In a small bowl or food processor, combine cream cheese, Parmesan cheese, lemon juice, and hot sauce. Blend well.
2. Cut smoked salmon into about 30 pieces. Spoon about 2 teaspoons of cheese mixture over pieces of salmon and top each with dill or parsley. Bake until cheese is softened, about 5 minutes. Serve warm.

COMPATIBLE with "B" and Neutral

*Optional for Working People: Same as Day One

DINNER:

Pizza Napoli

A&B Pizza Dough (see basic recipe, same as Day One or cookbook)
A&B Pizza Sauce (see basic recipe, same as Day One or cookbook)
1 1/2 cups feta, shredded
Olives (quantity to taste)
3 cups mozzarella, shredded

1. Prepare pizza dough.
2. Prepare pizza sauce.
3. Preheat oven to 350°F
4. Spread mixture evenly over dough. Top with feta and olives. Place baking sheet on lowest shelf in oven and bake until crust is firm and golden brown, 15 to 20 minutes. Serve warm.

COMPATIBLE with "A" and Neutral

OPTIONAL: Same as Day One

DAY NINETEEN

BREAKFAST:
Same as Day One

LUNCH:

Cauliflower Soufflé Côte d'Azur*   4 servings
1 large cauliflower (cored and broken into small florets)
3 tablespoons olive oil
2 egg yolks
1/2 cup parsley, chopped
1 pinch sweet Hungarian paprika (or other paprika)
1 pinch nutmeg

1. Preheat oven to 350°F.
2. In a saucepan, cook cauliflower in boiling salted water for 10 minutes. Remove from heat.
3. In a small soufflé dish, heat oil.
4. Whisk two egg yolks, with 3 teaspoons oil, nutmeg, pepper, and parsley.
5. Spread mixture over cauliflower. Bake until soufflé is golden brown, 10 minutes.

COMPATIBLE with "A", "B", and Neutral

*Optional for Working People: Same as Day One

DINNER:

Classic Roast Chicken   4 servings

1 whole chicken
1 medium onion, thickly sliced
1 small onion, diced
2 carrots, thickly sliced
2 zucchini, sliced
2 tablespoons butter
2 tablespoons olive oil
1 tablespoon soy flour
1 cup chicken stock or water
1 tablespoon dried thyme
Salt and pepper to taste

1. Rinse and dry the chicken.
2. Preheat oven to 350°F. Season chicken liberally with salt and pepper inside and out. Put small quartered onions and thyme inside cavity and tie legs together. Rub butter all over chicken.
3. Put oil in a large oval gratin dish or shallow roasting pan. Scatter sliced onions, zucchini, and carrots around the dish. Place chicken on top.
4. Roast chicken in oven until it is golden brown, about 20 minutes per pound.
5. Remove chicken to a serving platter and cover with foil to keep warm.
6. Remove all but 2 tablespoons fat from pan. Place over medium heat, add soy flour, and cook, stirring, until thickened. Season with salt and pepper to taste. Strain into a gravy boat and serve with chicken.

COMPATIBLE with "B" and Neutral

OPTIONAL: Same as Day One

DAY TWENTY

BREAKFAST:
Same as Day One

LUNCH:

Hawaiian Chicken Salad*   4 servings
1/2 pound cooked chicken (leftovers), diced
2 cups pineapple, diced
1 cup mayonnaise
Dash vinegar
Dash pepper
Pinch garlic salt
Pinch nutmeg

1. In a medium bowl, combine all ingredients; mix well.
2. Chill thoroughly. Serve on lettuce; top with diced pineapples.

COMPATIBLE with "B" and Neutral

*Optional for Working People: Same as Day One

DINNER:

Potato Salzburg with Sour Cream   4 servings

10 small new potatoes
1/2 cup sour cream
1/2 bunch chives, minced

1. Preheat oven to 400°F.
2. Arrange potatoes on a baking sheet. Bake potatoes until tender, about 40 minutes. Place potatoes in a large bowl. Let stand until potatoes are cool enough to handle.
3. Halve potatoes. Cut a thin slice from the rounded end of each potato half so it will stand upright. Using a small spoon, scoop out center from each potato half, leaving a shell about 1/4-inch.
4. Using a small spoon, fill each potato cavity with 2 teaspoons sour cream.
5. Cook until heated through, about 10 minutes. Garnish with chives

COMPATIBLE with "A" and Neutral

OPTIONAL: Same as Day One

DAY TWENTY-ONE

BREAKFAST:
Same as Day One

LUNCH:

A&B Power Salad*
(Same as Day One)

With anything from the Neutral group, "A", or "B"

*Optional for Working People: Same as Day One

DINNER:

Oriental Lentil Soup   4 servings
1 1/2 cups lentils
2 cups vegetable or chicken bouillon (or cubes)
8 cups (distilled) water
1 large onion, minced
1 clove garlic, crushed through a press
2 stalks celery, chopped
2 large carrots, chopped
2 tablespoons fresh parsley, chopped
1/2 teaspoon sea salt
1 teaspoon dried oregano
1 teaspoon sweet Hungarian paprika
1/2 teaspoon dried thyme
3 tablespoons olive oil

1. In a saucepan, melt oil over medium-high heat. Add onions, tossing for 5 minutes until crisp-tender.

2. Add garlic, carrots, and celery. Add seasonings and herbs; mix well, tossing for 3–4 minutes. Add vegetable or chicken bouillon; cook for 3 minutes.
3. Add lentils and 8 cups hot water. Simmer over low heat for 60 minutes.

COMPATIBLE with "A", "B", and Neutral

OPTIONAL: Same as Day One

DAY TWENTY-TWO

BREAKFAST:
Same as Day One

LUNCH:

Broccoli Milanese*   2 servings
4 stalks broccoli, washed & stems cut off
2 tablespoons butter
2 tablespoons fresh lemon juice
Seasoning to taste

1. Cut each broccoli stem into individual florets. Place in vegetable steamer over boiling water until tender, covered, for 7 minutes.
2. In a small saucepan, melt butter; mix with lemon juice. Pour sauce over hot broccoli. Season to taste.

COMPATIBLE with "A", "B", and Neutral

*Optional for Working People: Same as Day One

DINNER:

Swordfish Steak   4 servings

4 swordfish steaks, 4–6 ounces each
2 tablespoons grated Parmesan cheese
2 cloves garlic, peeled
1/3 cup olive oil
1/4 cup pine nuts
1 cup fresh basil leaves
1/4 teaspoon salt
1/8 teaspoon pepper
Lemon slices

1. Preheat oven to 425°F. Arrange fish steaks in a large, lightly oiled baking dish. In a food processor, combine basil, garlic, pine nuts, Parmesan cheese, salt, and pepper. Puree until smooth. With machine on, slowly pour in olive oil. Process until mixture is well blended.
2. Spread mixture evenly over swordfish steaks. Cover dish loosely with aluminum foil. Bake until steaks are white throughout but still moist, 10–12 minutes. Garnish with thin slices of lemon.

COMPATIBLE with "B" and Neutral

OPTIONAL: Same as Day One

DAY TWENTY-THREE

BREAKFAST:
Same as Day One

LUNCH:

Asparagus Salad*   2–3 servings
1 head lettuce
1/2 head red leaf lettuce
1/2 pound fresh (or canned) asparagus
3 tablespoons olive oil
1 tablespoon vinegar
1 clove garlic, crushed through a press
1/2 tablespoon mustard
Sea salt to taste
Fresh ground black pepper

1. Wash salad; dry and break into pieces. Break off and discard heavy ends from asparagus.
2. In a medium saucepan, cook asparagus in boiling salted water until tender, 3–5 minutes. Remove from water, drain well, and cut into 1 1/2-inch pieces. Combine with lettuce.
3. For dressing, combine oil, mustard, sea salt, and lemon juice (or vinegar) in cup. Add pepper to taste. Mix well. Pour over salad.

COMPATIBLE with "A", "B", and Neutral

*Optional for Working People: Same as Day One

DINNER:

French Cabbage Roll   4 servings
1 large white cabbage
2 pounds ground meat
1/2 pound mushrooms (optional)
2 whole eggs
1/2 cup sour cream
3 large onions, chopped
1 clove garlic, crushed through a press
4 tablespoons butter or olive oil
1 pinch thyme
1 pinch cumin and fennel seed

1 pinch pepper
1 pinch sweet Hungarian paprika (or other)
1 pinch sea salt

1. Place cabbage in a vegetable steamer for 5–7 minutes (or in boiling water). Cook until leaves are tender when pierced with tip of sharp knife. Separate tender leaves. Cut leaves in quarter.
2. In a small frying pan, cook onions until golden brown.
3. In a big bowl, combine ground meat, onions, eggs, and spices. Mix well.
4. On a big plate, arrange leaves and form mixture into balls. Arrange balls on prepared cabbage leaves. Wrap cabbage around meat. Bind it with cotton string.
5. In a large frying pan, melt 4 tablespoons of butter over medium heat. Add onions and cabbage rolls. Cook cabbage rolls, turning, until brown. When golden brown, add sour cream and 1/2 cup of water. Let stand on low heat, 45 minutes. Serve warm.

COMPATIBLE with "B" and Neutral

OPTIONAL: Same as Day One

DAY TWENTY-FOUR

BREAKFAST:
Same as Day One

LUNCH:

Swiss Cheese Salad* 2–3 servings
1/2 pound Swiss cheese, cut in thin 1/2-inch slices
2 medium onions, thinly sliced into rings
Olive oil to taste
Vinegar to taste
Salt to taste
Pepper to taste

In a medium bowl, combine all ingredients. Add salt and pepper to taste.
Mix well.

COMPATIBLE with "B" and Neutral

*Optional for Working People: Same as Day One

DINNER:

Pasta di Paesano 4 servings
1/2 pound elbow macaroni
Feta cheese (quantity to taste)
1 cup heavy cream
4 cloves garlic, crushed through a press
Fresh mint (quantity to taste), chopped
Fresh spinach (quantity to taste), chopped
Olive oil to taste

1. Combine fresh spinach, fresh mint, feta cheese, cream, olive oil and garlic; set aside.
2. In a saucepan, cook macaroni in boiling salted watcr until tender but firm. Remove from heat and drain. Add mixture to macaroni. Mix well.

COMPATIBLE with "A" and Neutral

OPTIONAL: Same as Day One

DAY TWENTY-FIVE

BREAKFAST:
Same as Day One

LUNCH:

Artichokes Venetian*   2 servings
4 artichokes
Several stalks celery
1 bay leaf
1 clove garlic, crushed through a press

1. Wash artichokes. Trim end of stems. Snip thorny tip off each leaf. Combine garlic, celery stalks, and bay leaf.
2. In a vegetable steamer, place artichokes over boiling water; steam for 30 to 40 minutes. As soon as leaves can be easily removed, discard bay leaf, celery and garlic. Serve with melted butter for dipping.

COMPATIBLE with "A", "B", and Neutral

*Optional for Working People: Same as Day One

DINNER:

Ramses Beans & Ramses Salad
(Same as Day Eleven)

PLAN AHEAD: Soaking of the beans requires 3 to 4 hours plus 4 to 5 hours of cooking time !

OPTIONAL: Same as Day One

DAY TWENTY-SIX

BREAKFAST:
Same as Day One

LUNCH:

Grilled Steak, Sausages and/or Hamburger with grilled tomatoes, onions, pepper, zucchini*

Serve with sour cream and oregano and thyme or any other dip (see recipe cookbook) and "B"-fruits.

COMPATIBLE with "B" and Neutral

*Optional for Working People: Same as Day One

DINNER:

A&B Power Salad
(Same as Day One)

With anything from the Neutral group, "A", or "B"

OPTIONAL: Same as Day One

DAY TWENTY-SEVEN

BREAKFAST:
Same as Day One

LUNCH:

Classic Potato Soup*   4 servings
8 potatoes (medium to large), chopped in cubes
6–7 cups (distilled) water
2 tablespoons butter
1 teaspoon olive oil
1 large onion, chopped
1 clove garlic, minced
2 cups celery, chopped
4 cups vegetable bouillon (optional: 4 bouillon cubes)
1/4 teaspoon dried tarragon
1/2 teaspoon dried sage
1 teaspoon dried thyme
1 dash cayenne pepper
1 dash nutmeg
1 dash sea salt

In a large saucepan, melt butter and heat oil. Add onion, garlic, celery, potatoes, and spices. Add bouillon to cover vegetables. Bring to a boil. Simmer until vegetables are soft, for 20 minutes. Mash vegetables and potatoes. Serve warm.

COMPATIBLE with "A" and Neutral

*Optional for Working People: Same as Day One

DINNER:

Chicken Nuggets   4 servings

2 1/2 pounds skinless, boneless chicken breasts cut into 1-inch pieces
Olive oil for frying
1/2 cup cream (with water)
1/4 cup soy flour
1/4 cup grated Parmesan cheese
1 teaspoon paprika
1/2 teaspoon oregano

1. In a large frying pan, heat 1 inch of oil to 350°F.
2. Meanwhile, put cream in a bowl. In a paper bag, combine flour, Parmesan cheese, paprika, and oregano. Mix well. First dip chicken pieces in cream; then place about a dozen pieces of chicken at a time in bag and shake to coat.
3. Fry chicken in hot oil in batches, turning occasionally, for about 5 minutes, until crisp and golden brown. Drain on paper towels; serve hot.

COMPATIBLE with "B" and Neutral

OPTIONAL: Same as Day One

DAY TWENTY-EIGHT

BREAKFAST:
Same as Day One

LUNCH:

Peking Chicken Salad*   4 servings
1 pound cooked (or fried) chicken, diced (or any kind of poultry)
2 oranges, diced (without seeds)
2 tablespoons grated orange peel
2 cups mayonnaise
1 cup almonds, cut in halves
Dash cognac
Pinch nutmeg

> In a large bowl, combine all ingredients and mix well. Chill thoroughly. Serve on lettuce; garnish with orange slices.

COMPATIBLE with "B" and Neutral

*Optional for Working People: Same as Day One

DINNER:

Pizza Romana

A&B Pizza Dough and A&B Pizza Sauce (see basic recipe Day One or cookbook)
1 large onion, sliced
1 large green pepper, sliced
1/2 pound mushrooms, sliced
2 cloves garlic, grated
1/2 pound leek, chopped
1/2 pound ewe's milk cheese
1 cup sour cream
1 tablespoon fresh basil, chopped (or 1 teaspoon dried)
Dried oregano to taste
1/2 pound olives (any kind)
3 cups mozzarella, shredded

1. Prepare pizza dough and pizza sauce.
2. Preheat oven to 350°F.
3. In a small bowl, steam onions tender but not brown. Add leek, 1 cup ewe's milk cheese, basil, and sour cream. Spread mixture evenly over dough.
4. Cut remaining ewe's milk cheese in cubes.
5. Top pizza with olives, pepper, onions, mushrooms, and ewe's milk cheese.
6. Sprinkle mozzarella and oregano over the pizza.
7. Bake on lowest shelf until crust is firm and golden brown at edges, 20–25 minutes. Cut into serving pieces and serve warm.

COMPATIBLE with "A" and Neutral

OPTIONAL: Same as Day One

Chapter 17

FOUR-WEEK EXAMPLE MENU
For People With Health Problems,
Weight Problems and/or Over 40

LEVEL TWO

The A&B LEVEL TWO Chart was designed specifically for anyone currently experiencing health or weight problems or happen to be over 40 years of age

LEVEL TWO was designed to help your BioChemical Machine build up its alkaline on a daily basis. You have to make up for those years, probably decades, when you unknowingly decreased your *alkaline reserves*. Fortunately, this task is easier than you might first think.

In order to make following the LEVEL TWO CHART easier, we prepared a second color-coded version of the LEVEL ONE A&B Chart.

The color-coding clarifies which food items are base-builders *(yellow)*, healthy "good" proteins *(yellow and white)*, and healthy carbohydrates *(yellow and white)*.

The healthy acid-builders are *white;* the "bad" proteins are highlighted in *gray,* and the "extreme-bad" proteins are *red.* The unhealthy denatured (new history) carbohydrates are also *gray.*

> *Discuss the A&B Method with your medical doctor. S/he will be happy to help you incorporate these principles into his/her prescribed treatment plan.*

Don't be surprised to see the A&B Power Salad and optional Ramses Salad throughout this four-week example menu. They each emphasize a variety of leafy greens in addition to raw cauliflower, broccoli, spinach, and cabbage. These are vegetables most of us are use to eating cooked. Eaten raw, these are the types of food your Biochemical Machine is yearning for*!*

- Cauliflower is high in pantothenic acid and is called the "rejuvenation vitamin." It demolishes fat and plays a central role in the biochemical reactions within the body.

- Broccoli is rich in vitamin B_6, which converts energy reserves into sugar and gives immediate strength. Broccoli is gifted with the power to detoxify and to strengthen the immune system, as well as preventing cancer.

- White and red cabbage is rich in vitamin B_6.

- Spinach is rich in vitamin B_2, which regulates fat metabolism and sugar metabolism.

Your first culinary experience with this "power bowl" of food - seasoned with mayonnaise, vinegar, oil, salt, pepper, and herbs or other dressing and dips - will delight your taste buds and invigorate your body chemistry!

I offer the following twelve points as an overview for helping you more easily adopt the LEVEL TWO principles:

(1) REMEMBER ESSENTIAL#1: Eat from group "A"—Eat group "B" but as much as possible AVOID eating from both at the same meal. Wait at least three hours before switching between "A" to "B" or vice versa. <u>Neutrals may be eaten at any time with no waiting period</u>.

(2) EAT SMART: The key to health and well-being is simple: <u>80%</u> of your daily intake of foods should be <u>base-builders</u> *(yellow),* i.e., all kinds of (fresh) vegetables, salads, fruits, nuts, and healthy carbohydrates, such as potatoes, kale, bananas, dates, figs, honey and healthy olive or flaxseed oils (ideally, virgin oils).

(3) EAT HEALTHY: The other <u>20%</u> should be <u>base-building</u> dairy products *(yellow)* or <u>healthy acid-builders</u>: Neutral dairy products *(white),* whole wheat products *(white),*

brown rice *(white)* or other Neutral foods—for example, legumes *(white,* correct preparation is vital!), Neutral meat *(white),* Neutral fish *(white),* or other foods that are *white* on the A&B Chart.

(4) THE KEY POINTS
- Vegetables, salads, and fruits should be eaten <u>FRESH</u>. Potatoes should be steamed in their skins.
- Variety is spice of life!
- Make the "A&B Power Salad" or optional Ramses Salad the foundation of your daily menu. See the four-week example menus and cookbook. The best vegetables for increasing alkaline are the root vegetables—raw carrots, turnips, beets, and all sorts of top vegetables such as spinach, sprouts, beet tops, chard, celery, onion tops, watercress, broccoli, cauliflower, or any green vegetable that contains juice.

(5) START YOUR DAY RIGHT: Begin your day with whole milk and two apples each morning. Apples and milk are extremely detoxifying. They keep sugar levels steady and help ensure that your Biochemical Machine obtains sufficient fiber, vitamins, and minerals. AVOID eating low-fat, fat-free, or skim milk products!

(6) AVOID "extreme-bad" proteins *(red)*, such as cooked meat and "bad" proteins *(gray)*, such as cooked fish, and cheese below 50% fat, as well as ready-made foods and any foods with artificial additives ("B"-column, *gray*).

(7) Try to replace "extreme-bad" proteins liked cooked meat and cooked fish with Neutral meat and fish.

(8) Although it is recommended you omit cooked meat (*red*) and cooked fish (*gray*) completely, sometimes there's nothing as tasty as a juicy steak. Strive to balance such meals with fresh base-building "B" and Neutral fruits to compensate for the poisonous debris of the "bad" and "extreme-bad" proteins.

(9) LIMIT, if not ELIMINATE all white flour products such as white bread, noodles, spaghetti, pasta, and white sugar. They are unhealthy acid-builders. Replace them with whole wheat products such as wheat bread and wheat noodles, which are healthy acid-builders. You may eat chocolate from time to time, also the A&B-Burger® but it must be eaten with compatible "A" and/or Neutral foods, never with "B."

(10) AVOID low-fat and fat-free products. They contain sugars and chemicals that wreak havoc with your BioChemical Machine.

(11) AVOID the low-fat, fat-free, and/or skim milk products that contain sugar and other additives, They prevent your BioChemical Machine from obtaining vital vitamins and minerals

(12) AVOID industrialized oil, margarine *(gray)*, and trans fat *(red)*. Replace them with healthy natural oils (olive oil, flaxseed oil) and butter *(yellow)*.

(13) AVOID alcoholic beverages like sweet wine, champagne, whiskey, rye, etc., BUT YOU MAY DRINK BEER (with "A" and/or Neutral, never with "B") and, moderately, red wine.

REMEMBER THE BIG SEVEN ESSENTIALS

DAY ONE

1. BREAKFAST:

Milk & Apple
1–2 (better two!) medium-size apples (6 oz = 250 g)
3–4 glasses of whole milk (1 glass 250 ml = 1/4 of daily requirement)

OPTIONAL: yogurt or buttermilk

2. BREAKFAST:

Cottage Cheese with 2 Tomatoes
(Sliced with a of pinch sea salt; quantity to taste while following doctor's advice)

OPTIONAL: Cottage cheese or mozzarella with any kind of "B"-fruits or any other Neutral cheese, such as goat's milk cheese (feta) with olives, or anything else from the Neutral group

LUNCH:

The A&B Power Salad, along with milk and apples, should be your number one food choice. The Power Salad is a must. The Power Salad can be eaten during the day with salami (be careful that the salami is not precooked), smoked ham, or any other smoked, dried, or cured meat or fish.

<u>From late afternoon on</u>, you can eat the Power Salad with potatoes, (natural) rice, (wheat) pasta, or wheat bread with butter or mayonnaise. If you eat the Power Salad with wheat bread, potatoes, rice, or wheat pasta, you may eat also bananas, grapes, figs, and dates, as well as raisins, nuts, and honey ("A"), and, of course, anything Neutral at any time.

You can add any other vegetables you want. Remember: variety is important! There is no limit to vegetables, salads, sprouts, and herbs. You don't need to add ALL of the following suggested vegetables to your Power Salad, but it would be great if you did. By eating so many different vegetables and salads, your metabolism has it all.

A&B Power Salad

Lettuce (romaine, iceberg, limestone, red leaf, watercress, or any other lettuce, broken into bite-size pieces)
Tomatoes, sliced or diced into cubes
Carrot, chopped or sliced, quantity to taste
1/2 onion, chopped
1/2 to 1 cucumber, sliced or diced into cubes
Parsley, chopped, quantity to taste
Chive, or any other herb, to taste
Sprouts/soy sprouts to taste
1/2 green or red pepper, sliced or diced into cubes
Olives, quantity to taste
White and/or red cabbage, chopped, quantity to taste
Cauliflower, florets, quantity to taste
Broccoli, florets, quantity to taste
Spinach, chopped, quantity to taste

1. Cut up vegetables, small or large to taste. In a large bowl, combine all vegetables.
2. In a small bowl, combine olive oil, apple vinegar, and sea salt. Pour over salad.

> **TIP FOR WORKING PEOPLE:**
> *Locate a local deli where you can compose your Power Salads. If there is no salad bar around, eat fruits and cottage cheese instead, and save the Power Salad for dinner.*

> **HELPFUL TIP**: *Most people quickly tire of cutting up vegetables day in and day out. In order to have this vital food available at any time, prepare a huge bowl of raw vegetables sufficient for a couple of days. Vegetables don't perish quickly and can be kept refrigerated for several days. Chop or slice carrots and white and/or red cabbage and prepare cauliflower and broccoli according to your taste. Put chopped onions in a separate bowl that can be closed, so that your refrigerator will not smell like onions! Prepare (wash and cut) only a limited amount of fresh leafy greens/lettuce, since those perish very quickly. When you come home, you just need to take a bit from every bowl and mix it with oil, vinegar and sea salt.*

AFTERNOON SNACK:

2 Medium Apples with any kind of cream cheese

OPTIONAL:
Any other "B"- or Neutral fruits with any kind of Neutral cheese
     OR
Goat's milk cheese (Feta) with olives or any other Neutral milk product.

LATER IN THE AFTERNOON:

<u>Smoked Whiting</u> with fresh lemon

<u>OPTIONAL</u>:
Raw carrots, dipped in olive or flaxseed oil
    OR
Cauliflower dipped in olive-oil/vinegar/sea-salt dressing

<u>OPTIONAL</u>:
A&B Sandwich (whole wheat roll with mayonnaise, tomatoes, salad, onions)
    OR
1 slice whole wheat bread with 1/2 oz butter,
1 medium tomato, sliced and 1 dash sea salt
    OR
2 oz rye-wheat or graham bread with any kind of cream cheese, and chives (or other herbs and vegetables), chopped, 1 pinch sea salt
    OR
1 slice whole wheat bread with 1/2 oz butter, and 1 1/2 oz cured ham, or beef-salami (may not be precooked!) i.e., any other Neutral meat

DINNER:

New Potatoes Marseilles*

5 small red-skinned (if possible, organic) potatoes, unpeeled
(Alternative: 1–2 New Jersey potatoes, russet potatoes, or any other type)
2–3 tablespoons butter, melted
1/4 cup fresh parsley, chopped
Sea salt to taste

1. In a vegetable steamer, bring water to a boil. Place washed potatoes over boiling water for 20 minutes. Cook until tender. Remove from heat. Place potatoes in a large bowl. Let stand until potatoes are cool enough to handle.
2. Cut unpeeled potatoes into 1/4-inch slices. Place on baking sheet, and sprinkle evenly with butter. Sprinkle with seasoning and place as close as possible to heat of broiler until crusty and golden, approximately 10 minutes.

(Note: With Carbohydrates Chewing is Key!)

*Refer to the next page for An IMPORTANT note about diabetes and carbohydrates.

LATER IN THE EVENING:

3 to 5 oz Banana (chew!)

OPTIONAL:
Any other "A"- and/or Neutral fruits
And/or 1/4 oz raisins
And/or almonds, brazil nuts *(yellow)*
And/or cashew, filberts, hazelnuts, walnuts, etc. *(white)*
And 3 tablespoons 100% natural honey

OPTIONAL:
Buttermilk or any other Neutral cream cheese and Neutral milk product

OPTIONAL:
Ricotta cheese, 3 tablespoons 100% natural honey (kills bacteria), and almonds

---

About Diabetes:
Diabetes is a disease that affects the way the body uses food. Normally, the body turns food into sugar for energy. Then, the blood carries this sugar to cells throughout the body. There, insulin, a hormone, helps turn sugar from food into energy for the body to work. But, when you have diabetes, something goes wrong. The body makes little or no insulin and can't get blood sugar into the cells. As a result, the body doesn't get the fuel it needs and blood sugar stays too high. However, the word "sugar" is misleading. As fat doesn't make fat, it is not the ordinary "sugar" that causes "sugar." Diabetes is the result of many years of abuse of your BioChemical Machine. That's why you have a very high blood sugar level after having eaten carbohydrates. The healthier you get the better your sugar level gets—because you are improving the ability of your BioChemical Machine to cope with carbohydrates. At the beginning, diabetics should eat potatoes and/or pizza moderately.

DAY TWO

1. BREAKFAST:
Same as Day One

2. BREAKFAST:
Same as Day One

LUNCH:
Same as Day One

AFTERNOON SNACK:
Same as Day One

LATER IN THE AFTERNOON:
Same as Day One

DINNER:

Ramses Salad with Whole Wheat Bread (or Wheat Pita Bread)

5–6 fresh hot peppers, such as jalapenos
2–3 large tomatoes
1 head of lettuce
6 large cloves of garlic
2 large onions
1 bunch cilantro
1 lemon, peeled
1 tablespoon coriander
1 tablespoon cumin
Sea salt to taste
1/2 cup apple vinegar
1/2 cup olive oil

1. In a food processor, combine all ingredients. Process until well blended to form a pulp.
2. Serve Ramses Salad in small bowls; top with olive oil. Serve with whole wheat bread or wheat pita bread.

HELPFUL TIP: *In a jar, put remaining (leftover) Ramses Salad. Cover with olive oil, 2 inches above pulp (for conservation). Refrigerate for later use.*

LATER IN THE EVENING:
Same as Day One

DAY THREE

1. BREAKFAST:
Same as Day One

2. BREAKFAST:

Mozzarella with Tomatoes   4 servings
2 large tomatoes, sliced
1 ball of mozzarella, sliced
Fresh basil, quantity to taste
Lemon
Olive oil or virgin
Sea salt

1. Cut tomatoes and mozzarella in thin slices. Arrange on a plate.
2. In a small bowl, combine lemon and oil. Pour mixture over mozzarella and tomatoes. Add sea salt to taste. Garnish with fresh basil.

LUNCH:
Same as Day One

AFTERNOON SNACK:
Same as Day One

LATER IN THE AFTERNOON:
Same as Day One

DINNER:

Broccoli Milanese with Potatoes 4 servings

Potatoes, unpeeled
4 stalks broccoli, washed and stems cut off
2 tablespoons butter
2 teaspoons fresh lemon
Sea salt to taste

1. In a vegetable steamer, place unpeeled potatoes over boiling water for 20 minutes. Cook until tender. Keep warm.
2. Cut each broccoli stem into individual florets. Place in vegetable steamer over boiling water until tender, covered for 7 minutes.
3. In a small saucepan, melt butter. Pour this over hot broccoli. Season with sea salt. Serve with (peeled) potatoes.

LATER IN THE EVENING:
Same as Day One

DAY FOUR

1. BREAKFAST:
Same as Day One

2. BREAKFAST:
Same as Day One

LUNCH:
Same as Day One

AFTERNOON SNACK:
Same as Day One

LATER IN THE AFTERNOON:
Same as Day One

DINNER:

New Potatoes Marseilles   4 servings

5 small red-skinned potatoes, unpeeled
(Alternative: 1–2 New Jersey potatoes,
russet potatoes, or any other type)
2–3 tablespoons butter, melted
1/4 cup fresh parsley, chopped
Sea salt to taste

1. In a vegetable steamer, bring water to a boil. Place washed potatoes over boiling water for 20 minutes. Cook until tender. Remove from heat. Place potatoes in a large bowl. Let stand until potatoes are cool enough to handle.
2. Cut unpeeled potatoes into 1/4-inch slices. Place on baking sheet and sprinkle evenly with butter. Sprinkle with seasoning and place as close as possible to heat of broiler until crusty and golden, approximately 10 minutes.

COMPATIBLE with "A" and Neutral

OPTIONAL: 1–2 slices wheat bread with fresh butter, bacon and/or cheese above 60% fat (cream cheese, Camembert, Brie, cottage cheese, etc.), with raw vegetables and/or mixed salads

COMPATIBLE with "A" and Neutral

LATER IN THE EVENING:
Same as Day One

DAY FIVE

1. BREAKFAST:
Same as Day One

2. BREAKFAST:
Same as Day One

LUNCH:
Same as Day One

AFTERNOON SNACK:
Same as Day One

LATER IN THE AFTERNOON:
Same as Day One

DINNER:

Village Salad

1 pkg. (8 oz) feta cheese, cut into chunks
2 medium tomatoes, cut into chunks
1 large cucumber, cut into chunks
1 medium red onion, cut into chunks
1/2 cup A&B dressing (olive oil, apple vinegar, sea salt)

Toss all ingredients. Serve with wheat bread.

LATER IN THE EVENING:
Same as Day One

DAY SIX

1. BREAKFAST:
Same as Day One

2. BREAKFAST:
Same as Day One

LUNCH:
Same as Day One

AFTERNOON SNACK:
Same as Day One

LATER IN THE AFTERNOON:
Same as Day One

DINNER:

Cauliflower Soufflé Côte d'Azur   4 servings
1 large cauliflower, cored and broken into small florets
3 tablespoons olive oil
2 egg yolks
1/4 cup parsley, chopped
1 pinch sweet Hungarian or other paprika
1 pinch nutmeg

1. Preheat oven to 350°F.
2. In a saucepan, cook cauliflower in boiling salted water until just tender, about 10 minutes. Remove from heat.
3. In a small soufflé dish, heat 1 tablespoon oil.
4. Whisk two egg yolks with 2 tablespoons oil, nutmeg, and parsley.
5. Transfer cauliflower to soufflé dish.
6. Spread mixture over cauliflower. Place in broiler until soufflé is golden brown, about 5–7 minutes.

COMPATIBLE with "A", "B", and Neutral

Note: Cauliflower (pantothenic acid) detoxifies cells and plays a vital role in the biochemical reactions within the body—and it creates new skin.

LATER IN THE EVENING:
Same as Day One

DAY SEVEN

1. BREAKFAST:
Same as Day One

2. BREAKFAST:
Same as Day One

LUNCH:
Same as Day One

AFTERNOON SNACK:
Same as Day One

LATER IN THE AFTERNOON:
Same as Day One

DINNER:

Cabbage Budapest with Steamed Potatoes 4 servings

1 white cabbage, sliced
1 pound onions, diced
2 cups vegetable broth (or bouillon cubes)
2 cups heavy cream
1 cup sour cream
2 tablespoons butter
Sea salt to taste
2 teaspoon Hungarian or other paprika
Soy sauce to taste
Potatoes, quantity to taste

1. For potatoes, see Day One.
2. In a large saucepan, sauté onions in butter until golden brown. Add vegetable broth or bouillon cubes and sea salt.
3. Place cabbage in saucepan and cook for 15–20 minutes.
4. Remove from heat and drain cabbage.
5. Combine heavy cream and sour cream with paprika and season to taste. Sprinkle mixture over cabbage. Let stand 10 minutes.
6. Serve cabbage with (peeled) potatoes.

LATER IN THE EVENING:
Same as Day One

DAY EIGHT

1. BREAKFAST:
Same as Day One

2. BREAKFAST
Same as Day One

LUNCH:
Same as Day One

AFTERNOON SNACK:
Same as Day One

LATER IN THE AFTERNOON:
Same as Day One

DINNER:

**DON'T FORGET TO LEAVE ADAQUATE TIME
TO PREPARE YOUR DINNER
Soaking of the beans requires 3 to 4 hours and an additional
4 to 5 hours for cooking!**

Ramses Beans and Ramses Salad
Old Egyptian recipe; beans should be eaten with Ramses Salad to ensure proper digestion. (Optional: onions, dressed with vinegar, sea salt, and cumin. Crush onions with your hand to enhance the flavor.)

2 pounds small fava beans
1 pound skinless fava beans
1 pound Garbanzo beans (chickpeas)
1/2 pound yellow lentils
1 large bulb of garlic, crushed through a press
1 tablespoon cumin
2 tablespoons dried coriander
Sea salt to taste

1. Wash beans and lentils separately. In a big bowl, put fava beans, skinless fava beans, and Garbanzo beans. Cover beans with plenty of (distilled) cold water. Soak beans for 3 to 4 hours. Remove from water.
2. In a large saucepan, bring water to a boil. Add fava beans and Garbanzo beans. Cover with water, 4 inches above. Reduce heat.
3. Check the water level every hour, adding water if necessary.
4. Simmer over medium-low heat for 4 to 5 hours, until soft. As soon as beans are soft, add lentils. Let cook, for 1 hour, until soft. Add garlic, cumin, coriander, and sea salt. Let stand for 30 minutes.
5. For Ramses Salad, see Day Two.
6. Serve warm; top the Ramses Beans with Ramses Salad.

OPTIONAL: Mash beans with mixer. Top with Ramses Salad.

HELPFUL TIP: *Ramses Beans leftovers can be stored in the freezer. Put small portions in bowls or plastic bags for later consumption. For RAMSES SALAD, see Day Two.*

LATER IN THE EVENING:
Same as Day One

DAY NINE

1. BREAKFAST:
Same as Day One

2. BREAKFAST:
Same as Day One

LUNCH:

Mozzarella with Tomatoes   4 servings
2 large tomatoes, sliced
1 ball of mozzarella, sliced
Fresh basil
Vinegar
Olive oil
Sea salt

1. Cut tomatoes and mozzarella in thin slices. Arrange on a plate.
2. In a small bowl, combine vinegar and oil. Pour mixture over mozzarella and tomatoes. Add sea salt to taste. Garnish with fresh basil.

AFTERNOON SNACK:
Same as Day One

LATER IN THE AFTERNOON:
Same as Day One

DINNER:

Eggplant Normandy 4 servings

2 large eggplants (or 4 small)
6 cloves garlic, crushed through a press
4 small onions, peeled
2 medium tomatoes, pureed
2 cups olive oil
1 bunch parsley, chopped
1 bunch cilantro, chopped
Sea salt
Celery salt

1. Preheat oven to 300°F.
2. With a sharp knife, remove stem head of eggplants. Cut eggplants in 1/2-inch slices.
3. Chop cilantro and parsley. Puree tomatoes. Add garlic. Mix well.
4. In a large saucepan, heat olive oil. Place eggplants in oil. Fry until brown.
5. On a baking sheet, place eggplant slices. Sprinkle them with tomato-cilantro-parsley mixture. Bake for 20 minutes, until crispy. Season to taste.

LATER IN THE EVENING:
Same as Day One

DAY TEN

1. BREAKFAST:
Same as Day One

2. BREAKFAST:
Same as Day One

LUNCH:
Same as Day One

AFTERNOON SNACK:
Same as Day On

LATER IN THE AFTERNOON:
Same as Day One

DINNER:

<u>Creamy Cauliflower Soup</u>   4 servings
6 cups (distilled) water
2 medium cauliflower, cored and coarsely chopped
1 onion, chopped
1 clove garlic, crushed through a press
2 tablespoons butter
1 tablespoon olive oil
2 stalks celery, chopped
8 scallions, chopped
2 tablespoons vegetable broth (or bouillon cubes)
1/8 teaspoon nutmeg
1 teaspoon dried basil
1/2 teaspoon dried thyme
1 teaspoon dried marjoram
1/2 teaspoon celery or sea salt
1/8 teaspoon of fresh ground black pepper

In a large saucepan, melt butter and heat oil. Add scallions, onions, garlic, cauliflower, and celery. Season with sea salt to taste. Cook over medium heat for several minutes, stirring frequently. Add water and bouillon; bring to a boil. Add basil, thyme, marjoram. Simmer, covered, over medium heat until cauliflower is tender, for 10–15 minutes. Remove cover and cool slightly. In blender, process until soup is smooth and creamy. Add nutmeg to taste.

LATER IN THE EVENING:
Same as Day One

DAY ELEVEN

1. BREAKFAST:
Same as Day One

2. BREAKFAST:
Same as Day One

LUNCH:
Same as Day One

AFTERNOON SNACK:
Same as Day One

LATER IN THE AFTERNOON:
Same as Day One

DINNER:

Mushrooms Lyon   2 servings
1/2 pound mushrooms
2 tablespoons butter
1 tablespoon fresh lemon juice
Dash sea salt
Dash garlic salt
Soy sauce

1.   Wash mushrooms; cut and discard ends from stems. Cut mushrooms into slices.
2.   In a saucepan, melt butter. Add mushrooms, tossing lightly in butter, until soft. Add lemon juice. Season to taste.

LATER IN THE EVENING:
Same as Day One

DAY TWELVE

1. BREAKFAST:
Same as Day One

2. BREAKFAST:
Same as Day One

LUNCH:
Same as Day One

AFTERNOON SNACK:
Same as Day One

LATER IN THE AFTERNOON:
Same as Day One

DINNER:

Potato Salad d'Alsace   4 servings

6 new potatoes, unpeeled
Beef salami (may not be precooked!), diced into cubes
(OPTIONAL: smoked fish), quantity to taste
1 fresh cucumber, sliced
1 large tomato, cut into small cubes
2 large pickles (sour or sweet dill), chopped into very thin slices
1/2 bunch chives, chopped
Scallions, to taste, chopped
1 onion, chopped
Mayonnaise and/or chunky Blue Cheese dressing to taste
Olive or any other natural oil to taste
Apple vinegar to taste
Sea salt to taste

1. In a vegetable steamer, place potatoes over boiling water for 20 to 30 minutes. Cook until tender. Remove from heat. Place potatoes in a large bowl. Let stand until potatoes are cool enough to handle. Peel potatoes. Cut potatoes into 1/2-inch cubes.
2. Add olive oil, apple vinegar, vegetables, cucumber, (not pre-cooked!) salami (or fish), and mayonnaise to potatoes. Mix well.

LATER IN THE EVENING:
Same as Day One

DAY THIRTEEN

1. BREAKFAST:
Same as Day One

2. BREAKFAST:
Same as Day One

LUNCH:
Same as Day One

AFTERNOON SNACK:
Same as Day One

LATER IN THE AFTERNOON:
Same as Day One

DINNER:
Same as Day Five (Village Salad)

LATER IN THE EVENING:
Same as Day One

DAY FOURTEEN

1. BREAKFAST:
Same as Day One

2. BREAKFAST:
Same as Day One

LUNCH:
Same as Day One

AFTERNOON SNACK:
Same as Day One

LATER IN THE AFTERNOON:
Same as Day One

DINNER:

A&B Pizza Four Seasons

2 cups whole wheat flour
1 tablespoon yeast
1/2 cup water
2 tablespoons olive oil
1 tablespoon butter
1 teaspoon sea salt
Broccoli, small pieces, quantity to taste
Cauliflower, quantity to taste
Mushrooms, sliced, quantity to taste
1/2 eggplant, sliced into 3/4 inch
1 large onion, sliced into rings
3 cloves garlic
Olives, quantity to taste
3 cups mozzarella, shredded
1 cup Ricotta cheese
1/2 cup heavy cream
1 teaspoon oregano, 1 teaspoon dried parsley, and 1 teaspoon basil

1. <u>A&B Pizza Sauce:</u> In a food processor, combine Ricotta cheese, garlic, cream, oregano, parsley, dried basil. Process until a paste forms. Slowly add olive oil; set aside.
2. <u>Pizza Dough:</u> In a medium mixing bowl, combine flour, yeast, olive oil, sea salt, and water. Stir mixture together; knead with your hands until dough is firm but moist. (If necessary, add more water, 1 tablespoon at a time.) Let dough rest for 1 hour.
3. Knead dough again with your hands. Cover and let rise for 20 minutes in a warm place.
4. Preheat oven to 350°F. Sprinkle whole wheat flour over greased baking sheet. Roll out dough and place on baking sheet. Spread pizza sauce evenly over dough. Top with broccoli, cauliflower, mushrooms, eggplant, onions, olives. Sprinkle mozzarella evenly over the pizza.
5. Place baking sheet on lowest shelf in oven (or the floor of a gas oven) and bake until crust is firm and nicely brown, 15–20 minutes. Serve warm.

LATER IN THE EVENING
Same as Day One

DAY FIFTEEN

1. BREAKFAST:
Same as Day One

2. BREAKFAST:
Same as Day One

LUNCH:
Same as Day One

AFTERNOON SNACK:
Same as Day One

LATER IN THE AFTERNOON:
Same as Day One

DINNER:

Austrian Baked Potatoes "Arnold"   4 servings

Potatoes, quantity to taste)
Butter (1 tablespoon for each potato)
Sour cream
Parsley and chives
Sea salt
Aluminum wrap

1. With a sharp knife, make a lengthwise cut across each potato. Season potatoes with sea salt to taste. Top each potato with a tablespoon of butter. Wrap each potato in aluminum wrap.
2. Preheat oven to 400°F. Place potatoes on baking sheet. Bake until tender, about 45 minutes.
3. In a bowl, mix sour cream with parsley and chives to taste. Serve warm (in aluminum wrap.)

LATER IN THE EVENING:
Same as Day One

DAY SIXTEEN

1. BREAKFAST:
Same as Day One

2. BREAKFAST:
Same as Day One

LUNCH:
Same as Day One

AFTERNOON SNACK:
Same as Day One

LATER IN THE AFTERNOON:
Same as Day One

DINNER:

<u>Italian Stuffed Green Peppers</u>   4 servings
1 cup natural (brown) rice
2 pounds mushrooms
2 middle-size onions, sliced
2 middle-size onions, cut in halves
8 green peppers (or 8 zucchini or 8 large tomatoes)
5 cloves garlic, crushed through a press (or garlic powder to taste)
1/2 bunch parsley, chopped
1/2 bunch cilantro, chopped
1/2 bunch dill, chopped
2 tablespoons butter or olive oil
1 large lemon, juice of
1 bouillon cube
1 pinch celery salt
1 pinch cumin
1 pinch saffron

1. In a small bowl, boil rice.
2. Cut mushrooms into small pieces.
3. Mix rice, mushrooms, parsley, cilantro, garlic and dill.
4. In a large bowl, combine vegetable, rice mix and seasonings (except saffron and lemon). Blend well.
5. With a sharp knife, cut off tops of green peppers (or tomatoes or zucchini). Carefully, remove seeds and veins, leaving stems intact.
6. Stuff vegetable with mixture.
7. Preheat oven to 350°F. In a large baking dish, melt 2 tablespoons of butter (or oil), bake 2 onions, cut in halves, until softened. Arrange vegetables.
8. In a small frying pan, heat 1 cup of water and add 1 bouillon cube, saffron, and lemon juice. Add to vegetables. Bake until vegetables absorb most of the juice. Remove from oven. Add sour cream. Let stand, 20 minutes. Serve warm.

LATER IN THE EVENING:
Same as Day One

DAY SEVENTEEN

1. BREAKFAST:
Same as Day One

2. BREAKFAST:
Same as Day One

LUNCH:
Same as Day One

AFTERNOON SNACK:
Same as Day One

LATER IN THE AFTERNOON:
Same as Day One

DINNER:
Same as Day Eight (Ramses Beans and Ramses Salad)
(OPTIONAL: Ramses Salad with Wheat Bread)

LATER IN THE EVENING:
Same as Day One

DAY EIGHTEEN

1. BREAKFAST:
Same as Day One

2. BREAKFAST:
Same as Day One

LUNCH:
Same as Day One

AFTERNOON SNACK:
Same as Day One

LATER IN THE AFTERNOON:
Same as Day One

DINNER:

Crispy Rice Balls St. Tropez   4 servings
1 cup brown rice
1 1/2 tablespoons butter
4 cups chicken broth (or bouillon)
Wheat or soy flour
3 egg yolks
1/4 pound mozzarella cheese, cut into small cubes
1/4 cup grated cheese (above 60% fat)
1/4 teaspoon grated nutmeg
1 tablespoon parsley, minced
Bread crumbs

1. In a medium saucepan, melt butter over medium-low heat. Add rice and cook, stirring, 2–3 minutes. Add 2 cups of broth (or bouillon). Cook rice, stirring 5–6 minutes. Add 1 more cup broth. Cook until fluid is almost absorbed, 4–5 minutes. Gradually add remaining broth. Cook, continuously stirring, until rice is tender but firm, about 10–15 minutes. Remove from heat. Let cool.
2. In a large bowl, beat 1 egg yolk. Add rice along with cheese, parsley, nutmeg. Blend well. Cover mixture and refrigerate at least 1 hour, until chilled.
3. After 1 hour, in a small bowl, beat 2 egg yolks with 2 teaspoons water; set aside.
4. Scoop mixture. Place mozzarella in center. Shape rice with the palms of your hands into balls (1 1/2 inches). Roll balls in flour. Roll balls in egg yolks. Coat balls with bread crumbs. Place rice balls on a baking sheet. Cover with plastic wrap. Refrigerate for 2 hours.
5. In a heavy saucepan, heat 3 inches of oil to 375°F; then add rice balls. Fry, occasionally turning, for 3–5 minutes, until golden brown. Remove with a slotted spoon. Drain on paper towels. Serve at once.

COMPATIBLE with "A" and Neutral

LATER IN THE EVENING:
Same as Day One

DAY NINETEEN

1. BREAKFAST:
Same as Day One

2. BREAKFAST:
Same as Day One

LUNCH:
Same as Day One

AFTERNOON SNACK:
Same as Day One

LATER IN THE AFTERNOON:
Same as Day One

DINNER:

Smoked Salmon and Feta Cheese   2 servings
3 ounces thinly sliced smoked salmon
1/4 teaspoon hot pepper sauce
Dash of lemon juice
8 ounces natural cream cheese, softened
1 cup fresh dill or parsley
3/4 cup grated Feta cheese (about 3 ounces)

1. Preheat oven to 400°F. In a small bowl or food processor, combine cream cheese, Feta cheese, lemon juice, and hot sauce. Blend well.
2. Cut smoked salmon into about 30 pieces. Spoon about 2 teaspoons of cheese mixture over pieces of salmon and top each with dill or parsley. Bake until cheese is softened, about 5 minutes. Serve warm.

LATER IN THE EVENING:
Same as Day One

DAY TWENTY

1. BREAKFAST
Same as Day One

2. BREAKFAST:
Same as Day One

LUNCH:
Same as Day One

AFTERNOON SNACK:
Same as Day One

LATER IN THE AFTERNOON:
Same as Day One

DINNER:

Cauliflower Soufflé Côte d'Azur   4 servings

1 large cauliflower (cored and broken into small florets)
3 tablespoons olive oil
2 egg yolks
1/4 cup parsley, chopped
1 pinch sweet Hungarian paprika (or other paprika)
1 pinch nutmeg

1. Preheat oven to 350°F.
2. In a saucepan, cook cauliflower in boiling salted water for 10 minutes. Remove from heat.
3. Place cauliflower in small soufflé dish.
4. Whisk two egg yolks, with olive oil, nutmeg, and parsley.
5. Combine egg mixture with cauliflower. Bake until soufflé is golden brown, 20 minutes.

LATER IN THE EVENING:
Same as Day One

DAY TWENTY-ONE

1. BREAKFAST:
Same as Day One

2. BREAKFAST:
Same as Day One

LUNCH:
Same as Day One

AFTERNOON SNACK:
Same as Day One

LATER IN THE AFTERNOON:
Same as Day One

DINNER:

Potato Salzburg with Sour Cream   4 servings
10 small new potatoes
1/2 cup sour cream
1/2 bunch chives, minced

1. Preheat oven to 400°F. Arrange potatoes on a baking sheet.
   Bake potatoes until tender, about 40 minutes. Place potatoes in a
   large bowl. Let stand until potatoes are cool enough to handle.
2. Halve potatoes. Cut a thin slice from the rounded end of each
   potato half, so it will stand upright. Using a small spoon, scoop
   out center from each potato half, leaving a shell about 1/4 inch.
   Using a small spoon, fill each potato cavity with 2 teaspoons
   sour cream. Cook until heated through, about 10 minutes.
   Garnish with chives.

LATER IN THE EVENING:
Same as Day One

DAY TWENTY-TWO

1. BREAKFAST:
Same as Day One

2. BREAKFAST:
Same as Day One

LUNCH:
Same as Day One

AFTERNOON SNACK:
Same as Day One

LATER IN THE AFTERNOON:
Same as Day One

DINNER:

Oriental Lentil Soup   4 servings

1 1/2 cups lentils
2 cups vegetable or chicken bouillon (or cubes)
8 cups (distilled) water
1 large onion, minced
1 clove garlic, crushed through a press
2 stalks celery, chopped
2 large carrots, chopped
2 tablespoons fresh parsley, chopped
1/2 teaspoon sea salt
1 teaspoon dried oregano
1 teaspoon sweet Hungarian paprika
1/2 teaspoon dried thyme
3 tablespoons olive oil

1. In a saucepan, melt olive oil over medium-high heat. Add onions, tossing for 5 minutes, until crisp-tender.
2. Add garlic, carrots, and celery. Add seasonings and herbs; mix well, tossing for 3–4 minutes.
3. Add vegetable or chicken bouillon; cook for 3 minutes.
4. Add lentils and 8 cups hot water. Simmer over low heat for 60 minutes.

LATER IN THE EVENING:
Same as Day One

DAY TWENTY-THREE

1. BREAKFAST:
Same as Day One

2. BREAKFAST:
Same as Day One

LUNCH:
Same as Day One

AFTERNOON SNACK:
Same as Day One

LATER IN THE AFTERNOON:
Same as Day One

DINNER:

Broccoli Milanese   2 servings
4 stalks broccoli, washed and stems cut off
2 tablespoons butter
2 tablespoons fresh lemon juice
Seasoning with sea salt, to taste

1. Cut each broccoli stem into individual florets. Place in vegetable steamer over boiling water until tender, covered, for 7 minutes.
2. In a small saucepan, melt butter and mix with lemon juice. Pour sauce over hot broccoli. Season to taste.

LATER IN THE EVENING:
Same as Day One

DAY TWENTY-FOUR

1. BREAKFAST:
Same as Day One

2. BREAKFAST:
Same as Day One

LUNCH:
Same as Day One

AFTERNOON SNACK:
Same as Day One

LATER IN THE AFTERNOON:
Same as Day One

DINNER:

Asparagus Salad   2–3 servings
1 head lettuce
1/2 head red leaf lettuce
1/2 pound fresh (or canned) asparagus
3 tablespoons olive oil
1 tablespoon apple vinegar or lemon juice
1 clove garlic, crushed through a press
1/2 tablespoon mustard
Sea salt to taste

1. Wash salad, dry, and break into pieces. Break off and discard heavy ends from asparagus.
2. In a medium saucepan, cook asparagus in boiling salted water until tender, 3–5 minutes. Remove from water, drain well, and cut into 1 1/2-inch pieces. Combine with lettuce.
3. For dressing, combine oil, garlic, mustard, sea salt, and lemon juice (or vinegar) in cup. Mix well. Pour over salad.

LATER IN THE EVENING:
Same as Day One

DAY TWENTY-FIVE

1. BREAKFAST:
Same as Day One

2. BREAKFAST:
Same as Day One

LUNCH:
Same as Day One

AFTERNOON SNACK:
Same as Day One

LATER IN THE AFTERNOON:
Same as Day One

DINNER:
Same as Day Eight (Ramses Beans and Ramses Salad)

LATER IN THE EVENING:
Same as Day One

DAY TWENTY-SIX

1. BREAKFAST:
Same as Day One

2. BREAKFAST:
Same as Day One

LUNCH:
Same as Day One

AFTERNOON SNACK:
Same as Day One

LATER IN THE AFTERNOON:
Same as Day One

DINNER:

Artichokes Venetian   4 servings
4 artichokes
Several stalks celery
1 bay leaf
1 clove garlic, crushed through a press

1. Wash artichokes. Trim end of stems. Snip thorny tip off each leaf. Combine garlic, celery stalks, and bay leaf.
2. In a vegetable steamer, place artichokes over boiling water; steam for 30–40 minutes. As soon as leaves can be easily removed, discard bay leaf, celery, and garlic. Serve with melted butter for dipping.

OPTIONAL:

Potato Soufflé   4 servings
4 large potatoes, steamed and 1/4-inch sliced
4 zucchini, 1/4-inch sliced
1 large onion, sliced
4 egg yolks
1/2 cup mozzarella, shredded
Herbs to taste
Fresh and/or dried parsley to taste
4 tablespoons butter or olive oil

1. In a vegetable steamer, place potatoes over boiling water, 20 minutes. Add zucchini. Cook until tender. Place potatoes in a large bowl. Let stand until potatoes are cool enough to handle. Peel and slice potatoes.
2. In a small bowl, whisk egg yolks. Add mozzarella. Mix well; set aside.
3. In a medium saucepan, cook onions in butter (or oil) until golden brown. Add potatoes and zucchini. Sprinkle mixture over potatoes and vegetables. Bake for another 3 minutes. Reduce heat. Cover saucepan. Let stand 15 minutes. Sprinkle herbs over soufflé.

LATER IN THE EVENING:
Same as Day One

DAY TWENTY-SEVEN

1. BREAKFAST:
Same as Day One

2. BREAKFAST:
Same as Day One

LUNCH:
Same as Day One

AFTERNOON SNACK:
Same as Day One

LATER IN THE AFTERNOON:
Same as Day One

DINNER:

Classic Potato Soup   4 servings
8 potatoes (medium to large), chopped into cubes
6–7 cups (distilled) water
2 tablespoons butter
1 teaspoon olive oil
1 large onion, chopped
1 clove garlic, minced
2 cups celery, chopped
4 cups vegetable bouillon (optional: 4 bouillon cubes)
1/4 teaspoon dried tarragon
1/2 teaspoon dried sage
1 teaspoon dried thyme
1 dash nutmeg
1 dash sea salt

In a large saucepan, melt butter and heat oil. Add onion, garlic, celery, potatoes, and spices. Add bouillon to cover vegetables. Bring to a boil. Simmer until vegetables are soft, for 20 minutes. Mash vegetables and potatoes. Serve warm.

LATER IN THE EVENING:
Same as Day One

DAY TWENTY-EIGHT

1. BREAKFAST:
Same as Day One

2. BREAKFAST:
Same as Day One

LUNCH:
Same as Day One

AFTERNOON SNACK:
Same as Day One

LATER IN THE AFTERNOON:
Same as Day One

DINNER:

Pizza Romana

Pizza Dough and Pizza Sauce (see basic recipe cookbook)
1 large onion, sliced
1 tablespoon olive oil
1 large green pepper, sliced
1/2 pound mushrooms, sliced
2 cloves garlic, grated
1/2 pound leeks, chopped
1/2 pound ewe's milk cheese
1 cup sour cream
1 tablespoon fresh basil, chopped (or 1 teaspoon dried)
Dried oregano to taste
1/2 pound olives (any kind)
3 cups mozzarella, shredded

1. Prepare Pizza Dough and A&B Pizza Sauce.
2. Preheat oven to 350°F.
3. In a small saucepan, sauté onions in olive oil until tender but not brown. Add leeks, 1 cup ewe's milk cheese, basil, and sour cream.
4. Spread mixture evenly over dough. Cut remaining ewe's milk cheese in cubes. Top pizza with olives, pepper, onions, mushrooms, and ewe's milk cheese. Sprinkle mozzarella and oregano over pizza. Bake on lowest shelf until crust is firm and nicely brown at edges, 20–25 minutes. Cut into serving pieces and serve warm.

LATER IN THE EVENING:
Same as Day One

PART VII

QUICK SOLUTION

Chapter 18

THE A&B TEN-DAY EXAMPLE
For Quick Weight Loss

Holy Cow! Look what makes you thin. . . .Grapefruit doesn't really rev up your metabolism. Cabbage doesn't really light a fuse under stored calories. But milk will. This isn't a new food fad; this is science. Just ask Michael Zemel, chairman of the nutrition department at the University of Tennessee in Knoxville. He's found that milk turns down the tendency of your fat cells to store the day's calories, and increases the amount frittered away as heat. . . .
Readers Digest, July 2002, page 107 by Lisa Davis.

- Whole milk and apples along with the A&B Power Salad or the optional Ramses Salad is the foundation of the A&B 10-Day Quick Loss Program. For those who lack patience and want—for whatever reasons—to lose weight quickly, these foods make the process both healthy and easy!

- BETWEEN MEALS eat Neutrals such as nuts (but no "A"-peanuts) and seeds, cooked egg yolks (without the whites), and/or raw cauliflower, tomatoes or any vegetable dipped in mayonnaise, salad dressing, olive oil, apple vinegar, sea salt, pepper, cottage cheese, goat's cheese, or any other Neutral cheese along with any Neutral meat or fish.

- BE CAREFUL with "B"-sausages! They are not pure meat but contain stuffing that will upset your chemistry. This will ultimately lead to weight gain.

- ELIMINATE any LOW-FAT or FAT-FREE products containing sugar and artificial additives. These chemicals interfere with your body's chemistry, the A&B principles and food chemistry.

- DRINK (distilled) water or tea with cream. Avoid sodas, even those without sugar.

- IF YOU FIND YOURSELF GETTING HUNGRY during the day, eat milk and apples because a well-balanced blood sugar level curbs your appetite.

DAY ONE

BREAKFAST:

Whole Milk & Apples
(Quantity to taste)

LUNCH:

Mozzarella with Tomatoes*   2 servings
2 large tomatoes, sliced
1 mozzarella, sliced
Fresh basil
Olive oil
Apple vinegar
Sea salt and pepper to taste

1. Cut tomatoes and mozzarella in slices. Arrange on a plate.
2. In a small bowl, combine vinegar and oil. Pour mixture over mozzarella and tomatoes. Add salt and pepper to taste. Garnish with fresh basil.

---

*OPTIONAL: *At work you may prefer to bring your food from home. Be sure to pack plenty of fruits from the "B" group - preferably apples - or any kind of salad similar to the A&B Power Salad. You can eat your salads and fruits with cottage cheese, goat or ewe's milk cheese, feta, mozzarella, cream cheese, Roquefort, ricotta, or anything from the Neutral group.*

> **IF YOU GET HUNGRY later during the day eat WHOLE MILK and APPLES because a well-balanced blood sugar level curbs your appetite!**

DINNER:

There is no limit to the quantity of vegetables, salads, sprouts, and herbs you may eat. Your salads don't need ALL of the following ingredients just keep in mind, variety is important! Eating so many different vegetables and salads will keep your BioChemical Machine happy and healthy.

A&B Power Salad with Goat's Cheese (or any other Neutral cheese)

Lettuce (romaine, iceberg, limestone, red leaf, watercress, or any other lettuce, broken into bite-size pieces)
Tomatoes, sliced or diced into cubes
Cucumber, sliced or diced into cubes
Carrots, chopped or sliced
Cauliflower, chopped
Broccoli, chopped
White and/or red cabbage, chopped
Sprouts/soy sprouts
Spinach, chopped
Onions, sliced or diced into cubes
Scallions, sliced
Parsley, chopped
Chive, chopped
Oil to taste (olive, flaxseed, sesame, etc.)
Apple vinegar (opt: Balsamic) or fresh lemon juice to taste
Salt (sea salt, herb salt, Bio-salt) to taste
Pepper to taste

1. Cut vegetables. In a large bowl, combine all vegetables.
2. In a small bowl, combine oil, vinegar, salt, pepper, and chives. Pour over salad.

DAY TWO

BREAKFAST:
Same as Day One

LUNCH:

Broccoli Milanese*   2–3 servings
4 stalks broccoli, washed and stems cut off
2 tablespoons butter
2 teaspoons fresh lemon juice
Seasoning to taste

1. Cut each broccoli stem into individual florets. Place in vegetable steamer over boiling water until tender, covered, for 7 minutes.
2. In a small saucepan, melt butter; combine with lemon juice. Pour sauce over hot broccoli. Season to taste.

*Optional for Working People: Same as Day One

IF YOU ARE GETTING HUNGRY . . .
eat whole milk and apples.

DINNER:

A&B Power Salad
(Same as Day One)

DAY THREE

BREAKFAST:
Same as Day One

LUNCH:

Cauliflower Soufflé Côte d'Azur*   4 servings
1 large cauliflower, cored and broken into small florets
3 tablespoons oil
2 egg yolks
1/4 cup parsley, chopped
1 pinch sweet Hungarian or other paprika
1 pinch nutmeg

1. In a saucepan, cook cauliflower in boiling salted water for 10 minutes. Remove from heat.
2. Whisk two egg yolks, with 3 teaspoons oil, nutmeg, pepper, and parsley together.
3. Preheat oven to 350°F. Spread mixture over cauliflower. Bake until soufflé is golden brown, about 10 minutes.

*Optional for Working People: Same as Day One

Note: *Cauliflower (which contains pantothenic acid) detoxifies cells and plays a vital role in the biochemical reactions within the body—and it creates new skin.*

IF YOU ARE GETTING HUNGRY . . .
eat whole milk and apples.

DINNER:

<u>A&B Power Salad</u>
(Same as Day One)

DAY FOUR

BREAKFAST:
Same as Day One

LUNCH:

<u>Sylvia's Tuna Salad</u>*   4 servings
1 (6 1/2 ounce) can tuna (in oil or water)
1/4 cup capers, cut in halves
2 tablespoons onions, chopped
2 tablespoons mustard
1/2 cup pickled dill or sweet cucumber, diced
1/3 cup parsley, chopped
Olive oil, quantity to taste
1 teaspoon fresh lemon juice (or apple vinegar)
1/4 teaspoon pepper
Sea salt to taste
Garlic salt to taste

In a medium bowl, mash tuna with oil and mustard. Add onions, lemon juice, pickled cucumber, capers, salt and pepper. Mix well. Serve on lettuce. Garnish with remaining capers or pickled cucumber slices.

*Optional for Working People: Same as Day One

DINNER:

<u>A&B Power Salad</u>
(Same as Day One)

DAY FIVE

BREAKFAST:
Same as Day One

LUNCH:

<u>Roast Chicken Hawaii</u>*   4 servings
1 whole chicken, about 3 pounds
2 tablespoons butter
2 tablespoons olive oil
1 cup pineapple, diced
1 teaspoon dried thyme
Sea salt and pepper to taste

1. Preheat oven to 350°F. Season chicken inside and out with salt and pepper. Place 1/2 teaspoon thyme in cavity. Tie legs together and rub butter over skin. Place in a large roasting pan.
2. Roast chicken for 15 minutes. Arrange diced pineapple around chicken. Sprinkle remaining thyme over chicken. Pour dry white wine over all and bake 1 hour and 15 minutes. Add water (or cream) as soon as wine evaporates.

*Optional for Working People: Same as Day One or fried chicken.

IF YOU ARE GETTING HUNGRY . . .
eat whole milk and apples.

DINNER:

<u>A&B Power Salad</u>
(Same as Day One)

DAY SIX

BREAKFAST:
Same as Day One

LUNCH:

<u>Mozzarella with Tomatoes*</u>   2–4 servings
2 large tomatoes, sliced
1 pound mozzarella, sliced
Fresh basil
Apple vinegar to taste
Olive oil to taste
Sea salt to taste
Pepper to taste

1. Cut tomatoes and mozzarella in thin slices. Arrange on a plate.
2. In a small bowl, combine vinegar and oil. Pour mixture over mozzarella and tomatoes. Add salt and pepper to taste. Garnish with fresh basil.

*Optional for Working People: Same as Day One
IF YOU ARE GETTING HUNGRY . . .
eat whole milk and apples.

DINNER:

A&B Power Salad
(Same as Day One)

DAY SEVEN

BREAKFAST:
Same as Day One

LUNCH:

Meatballs*   4 servings
2 pounds ground meat
2 onions, chopped
2 onions, sliced
2 celery stalks
3–4 cloves garlic
1/2 bunch parsley
1 large can Italian peeled tomatoes
Butter to taste
Soy sauce to taste
Sea salt to taste
Pepper to taste
Celery salt, oregano, basil to taste

1. In a food processor or blender, combine chopped onions, celery stalks, garlic, parsley, salt, pepper, celery salt, oregano, and basil. Process vegetables. Add meat and spices. Process until a puree forms. Form meatballs.
2. In a frying pan, combine butter and sliced onions until lightly brown. Add salt, pepper, oregano, parsley, celery salt, and basil.

Mix well. Add Italian peeled tomatoes; chop while cooking. Add meatballs and cook (low), turning, about 1 hour. Add soy sauce to taste.

*Optional for Working People: Same as Day One

IF YOU ARE GETTING HUNGRY . . .
eat whole milk and apples.

DINNER:

A&B Power Salad
(Same as Day One)

DAY EIGHT

BREAKFAST:
Same as Day One

LUNCH:

Mushrooms Lyon*   2–3 servings
1/2 pound mushrooms
2 tablespoons butter
1 tablespoon fresh lemon juice
Dash sea salt
Dash garlic salt
Soy sauce

1. Wash mushrooms; cut ends from stems. Cut mushrooms into slices.
2. In a saucepan, melt butter. Add mushrooms, tossing lightly in butter until soft. Add lemon juice. Season to taste.

*Optional for Working People: Same as Day One

IF YOU ARE GETTING HUNGRY . . .
eat whole milk and apples.

DINNER:

A&B Power Salad
(Same as Day One)

DAY NINE

BREAKFAST:
Same as Day One

LUNCH:

Mozzarella and Tomatoes*
(Same as Day One)

*Optional for Working People: Same as Day One

IF YOU ARE GETTING HUNGRY ...
eat whole milk and apples.

DINNER:

Chef Salad
Lettuce (quantity to taste)
Tomatoes, sliced or diced into cubes
Cucumbers, thinly sliced
Broccoli, sliced
Cauliflower, sliced
Carrots, thinly sliced
Onions, sliced or diced into cubes
1–2 boiled whole eggs, sliced
Swiss cheese, thinly sliced
Smoked ham, sliced
Cooked turkey or chicken, rectangular slices
Oil to taste
Apple vinegar to taste
Salt to taste
Pepper to taste
Mayonnaise (OPTIONAL: dip or salad dressing)

Cut up vegetables. In a large bowl, combine all vegetables, smoked and/or cooked ham, cooked turkey, or chicken. Add oil, vinegar, salt, and pepper. Add mayonnaise, dip, or dressing.

DAY TEN

BREAKFAST:
Same as Day One

LUNCH:

Swiss Cheese Salad*   2–3 servings
1/2 pound Swiss cheese, thinly sliced
2 medium onions, thinly sliced into rings
Olive oil to taste
Apple vinegar to taste
Salt to taste
Pepper to taste

In a medium bowl, combine all ingredients. Add salt and pepper to taste.
Mix well.

*Optional for Working People: Same as Day One

IF YOU ARE GETTING HUNGRY . . .
eat whole milk and apples.

DINNER:

A&B Power Salad
(Same as Day One)

PART VIII

PRACTICAL TIPS

Chapter 19

PRACTICAL TIPS:
From Parties to Fast Food Restaurants

The advantage of the A&B is that you can live and eat normally, regardless of whether you are in the first phase of recovering or have already recouped and are sticking to the A&B Method of eating. It is easy while shopping in the supermarket or attending parties, weddings, or birthday celebrations. It is easy in restaurants or while traveling. Even fast food restaurants, with their seductive foods, provide enough choices for you to be loyal to the program, to yourself, and to the laws of your body's chemistry. Even if you do eat chemically wrong—it's not the end of the world. Simply return to the A&B Method and soon you will be back on track.

At the start, before you know the A&B chart by heart, I suggest you keep it handy. A quick glance will help you properly negotiate the "pitfalls" at any party and therefore enable you to enjoy yourself.

Parties, Cookouts, Weddings

Don't listen to silly advice. Recently I heard one so-called diet expert recommend eating a yogurt *before* going to a party. This is utter nonsense. There are always plenty of good food choices at any party. What kind of logic is it that promotes eating before an eating event? I myself prefer to eat correctly at the event. However, if you are inclined to eat before going to a party, eat salads and/or vegetables. These foods will biochemically match anything you might savor at the party.

Since most people drink wine at dinner parties, I suggest choosing foods from the "B" group and, of course, Neutrals. This means meatballs with tomato sauce; sausages with tomato sauce; roast beef with salad dressing; Swiss cheese; Gouda and other cheeses (mostly below 50% fat); any kind of fruit except for bananas, grapes, figs, and dates; roast venison with cranberry; and salmon with horseradish sauce.

Chicken is often served at parties. If this is your choice, make sure it hasn't been fried with honey-dipped batter. If this is the case, then simply remove the skin and eat the chicken with mixed salads. You might also find rolled ham, salami, smoked sausages, smoked mackerel, smoked salmon (with horseradish and lemon), herring, and trout. These are fine with salad dressing, pickles, and pickled cucumbers. And, of course, any vegetable or salad with vinegar, oil, and salt is all right.

Potato and pasta salads made with peas, onions, chives, and mayonnaise are often served at parties. If these salads contain pieces of sausages, pass them by.

Salads with vinegar, oil, or mayonnaise are ok. Even if you choose to eat bread, you can eat it with butter, vegetables, and salads—and, of course, salad dressing. If there are cooked eggs, then eat only the egg yolk and crumble it on the bread with a bit of salt. It tastes better than you might expect. Egg yolk with salad dressing is also a tasty choice. If you choose bread, potatoes, and noodles, drink beer or sweet wine instead of dry wine and champagne.

If a cookout is on the horizon, you will have to make a choice: either corn with butter and salads *or* meat, such as hamburger, spare ribs, and sausages. If the spare ribs are coated with honey glaze, go ahead, eat them and simply return to the A&B Method the following day. After all, sometimes we all need to indulge a little. That next day, simply eat plenty of fruits, salads, and vegetables. Remember, even if you commit some "chemical mistakes," you can balance them the day after without any lasting problems.

Restaurants

Eating in restaurants is fairly easy. If you choose a full meal, you simply need to omit some food items. If you base your dinner on "B," you can start it with an hors d'oeuvre, such as mozzarella on tomatoes with vinegar, oil, and herbs; artichokes with dressing; eggplant with sour cream; smoked herring, salmon, or mackerel; or smoked ham or bacon (all Neutrals). Then you can continue, for example, with a steak topped with sour cream or herb butter; baked tomato; broccoli, green beans and peas (or other vegetables except kale, which is "A,") and for dessert, strawberries with whipped cream). Omit rice, potatoes, and bread. This is equally valid for chicken, turkey, goose, duck, or lamb chops. If the duck or chicken is baked with honey, don't eat the skin.

However, a small problem is presented if your meal included gravy made with flour. If this is the case, you will see it reflected on the scale the very next day. But again, this is just a small set back. Come back to this program the next day and your chemistry will begin to regulate itself once again. After a dinner that is based on "B," you can eat any kind of "B"-fruits, such as grapes, apples, oranges, or peaches, but not bananas ("A").

If you choose to eat your dinner based on "A" foods, such as spaghetti, rigatoni, or other pasta, instead of meat or fish, don't eat it with cooked tomatoes and/or ground meat. But you can eat it with cream, peas, mushrooms, or onions. You will see how good it tastes. Moreover, you will realize how good you feel after such a meal. For an hors d'oeuvre with a meal based on "A," try some goat or sheep's milk cheese with olives and salads or mozzarella with tomatoes, vinegar, oil, salt, pepper, and herbs. Or you can choose bread with Camembert or salami with mixed salad. You can also enjoy either potato or cauliflower soup.

The same applies if you eat baked potatoes with cottage or sour cream and chives, salads, and vegetables. As a dessert, you can eat banana flambé, cream cheese with raisins, or figs and dates, but no apples, strawberries, or other "B"-fruits.

Eating in a JAPANESE RESTAURANTS is easy. They offer a lot of Neutral *raw fish* such as sushi.

Fast Food Restaurants

Eating right in fast food restaurants is generally a bit more difficult. The most common foods, *sandwiches,* are made with rolls ("A"): roll with hamburger, roll with chicken, roll with roast beef, or roll with fish. Moreover, the sandwich or burger will be served with ketchup (cooked tomatoes, strong acid-builder "B") and french fries ("A"). If you have children, you will likely be unable to avoid fast food restaurants. We should admit that fast food really does taste seductively good, *yet you can still do it right:*

- In most restaurants you can order a sandwich with fresh tomatoes, lettuce, onions (or other vegetables), and mayonnaise (and skip the meat and ketchup).

- OR you could eat the sandwich (and french fries or onion rings) without the meat—which you could eat three hours later, at home.

- You can also eat only french fries or onion rings with salads ("A" and Neutral) and salad dressing, such as oil and vinegar.

- OR you can eat the other way around: hamburger (or other cooked meat) with ketchup and all kind of Neutral salads.

If you can find fast food restaurants that offer *pitas*, it will make your life easier because these breads are often stuffed with vegetables and mayonnaise (without chicken or other meat). And this is, of course, perfect.

Keep in mind that mayonnaise is Neutral.

Also, there is nothing wrong with a bagel and cream cheese in the morning (remember: don't prepare your coffee with milk—instead, use diluted cream).

Others, who follow this program to maintain their weight, can make individual modifications.

The milk shake can be temporary trouble. It contains milk, sometimes fruit from "B" *and* sugar, "A." However, even if you do succumb to this tasty delight, you can indulge in the salad bar to balance the meal.

Just in case you can't resist and end up eating the entire hamburger—bun and all—("A," "B," and Neutral), simply return to the A&B Method as soon as you are able.

A *hot dog* on a bun is probably the most difficult item, not only because this is clearly matching "A" with "B," but also, even if you omit the roll and eat only the frankfurter with mustard, it's not plain meat. Like other sausages, it contains additives, flour, and sugar and as such, it will put on the quick pounds. If you indulge in a hot dog from time to time, just get beck to the program as soon as possible. **NOTE: If you are in the process of curing or recovering from a disease, you shouldn't be eating this type acid-builders at all.**

One of the most popular fast foods is pizza. There are so many choices! Pizza with broccoli, mushrooms, onions, peppers, and olives tastes great and they are all chemically perfect. However, pay careful attention to the cheese. You should order the Neutral cheeses like mozzarella and other cheeses above 60% fat rather than the acid-building, Parmesan. Keep in mind that pizza dough is often made from white flour.

Therefore, avoid pizzas made with tomato sauce ("B"), since the white flour pizza dough is an "A."

Falafel is easy to eat. Unfortunately, it can be hard to find. It is made from flour and beans and can be eaten as offered. It's great with salads. Egyptians always eat beans with onions and radishes (base-builders). That's why they have so few problems digesting beans.

Chinese take-out is also easy because you can eat the meat or fish and vegetables without rice. Or you can eat just the rice with vegetables and no meat.

Be advised, since most Chinese restaurants put flour in their gravies, sugars in their sweet and sour sauces and serve white polished rice, added body weight can't be far behind.

Doughnuts can be eaten on the A&B Method, but eating them makes maintaining your weight and avoiding health problems a bit of a challenge. Doughnuts not only include acid-building sugar and white flour but also include ingredients such as milk and eggs. If you eat doughnuts from time to time, remember the three to four-hour waiting period and don't drink your coffee with milk but, instead, use diluted cream.

Pancakes in a restaurant are usually made from flour (buckwheat, white or whole wheat, all "A") and whole eggs "B" and therefore are in conflict. However, if you cannot resist, eat them with toppings like honey, bananas, raisins, dates, figs, dried apples, or plums, but NOT with "B"-fruits. *At home,* however, you can make them chemically correct ("Honey Pancakes," see The A&B Cookbook recipe). Remember the three to four-hour waiting period and don't eat them too often or you will see it on the scale.

Travel

It is just as easy to eat well on an airplane as it is in a restaurant. Airlines typically serve meat with vegetables and "B" (or Neutral) fruits. Simply avoid eating the breads, potatoes, rice and cookies. Or you can follow the reverse. Eat everything, including "A" and/or Neutral fruits and leave behind the cooked meats and fish.

It is important to avoid drinking alcohol. Instead, drink a *liter of water* each hour during your flight. Commercial airliners recycle cabin air in an attempt to conserve fuel, and the little fresh air they bring in is from high altitudes, where it is very dry.

If you are traveling in Europe, it's easy to follow the A&B Method. In France, Germany, Italy, Spain or Scandinavia you will have no problems. Even in places like Egypt you will find following the A&B Method easy. They offer great vegetables with meat and exotic seasoning. You will find fruits as sweet as you have never tasted. Wherever you go in this world you will find chemically matched foods for healthy eating.

Snacking

The healthiest snacking comes from anything within the Neutral column. No waiting periods and best of all, these foods can be eaten at any time. Almost all supermarkets are rich with selections of salads and vegetables, from mushrooms to beets, and lettuce to olives. Goat's milk or sheep's milk cheese is fine at any time because they too are Neutral.

If you want to have something between meals, stick to Neutrals since they may be eaten 24 hours a day, 7 days a week without complication. Of course, the best would be if you ate raw vegetables, salads and/or nuts. For example, a couple stalks of raw cauliflower dipped in a FRESH chunky blue cheese dressing made without preservatives.

In case you want to eat fruits, don't forget the waiting period of three to four hours if your next meal will include food from the "other" group or you intend to eat soon. Keep in mind that some fruits belong to "B," other fruits to "A," and blueberries, avocados and olives are Neutral.

If you eat carrots, don't forget to dip them in oil to make the vitamin A more readily available to your body.

Walnuts, hazelnuts, almonds, pistachios, cashews, and many other nuts are all Neutrals and great for snacking. But remember that peanuts belong to the "A" group. If you eat nuts (except peanuts) in the afternoon, and you would like to add them later in the evening, to a dessert, there is no need for any waiting period. They are all Neutral.

But if you eat nuts together with raisins ("A"), you should maintain the three to four hour waiting period in case you are invited for lunch or dinner where you might be served steak, turkey, or other meat or fish.

Other snacks, like *potato chips, pretzels,* or *flat breads,* need to be handled the same way. You eat them like every food from "A" and keep the waiting period in mind before switching to "B" foods.

Shopping

You don't need to buy your foods for the A&B Method in specialty or "health-food" stores. You just need to choose the right foods according to your body's chemistry not according to the gurus. Then, you are assured of eating healthfully. You can achieve this goal with foods readily available at your favorite supermarket. However,

(1) Don't buy low-fat or fat-free products, because they typically contain sugar, corn and plenty of additives to make them "tasty." The sugar will disturb your body's chemistry—and many important vitamins and minerals are absent from these items.

(2) Avoid buying prepared foods. They are full of chemicals, flour and sugars that will upset your body chemistry.

(3) If you buy canned foods, check the labels. If there is too much sugar in a product, avoid it. If you can make your own mayonnaise (see A&B Cookbook) at home, than do it.

(4) Buy whole wheat, rye, or other whole grain bread instead of white bread. Remember, the vitamins from the grain are removed from white bread. The price difference is extremely small and you will automatically eat less because your system is satisfied. Place the bread in your refrigerator to keep it fresh.

(5) Wash vegetables and fruits with warm water to remove as many pesticides (poisons) as possible. Don't forget that these dangerous chemicals are intended to kill animals and insects and some are extremely resistant.

(6) Organic foods (biological/ecological agriculture), such as vegetables and fruits, are good because you theoretically avoid pesticides and other poisons. Supermarkets increasingly are offering organic foods. But be careful when shopping for organic foods. Since they have yet to be regulated, some companies get away with selling non-organic foods at "organic" prices.

Cooking

When cooking, you should keep a copy of the A&B Chart close at hand. After deciding what to prepare, verify that all the ingredients fit together chemically. **This program is NOT about deprivation or quantity but about basic chemical principles**.

- Beware when recipes call for white flour. Use whole wheat flour or soy flour (Neutrals) when preparing foods from "B."

- Don't cook your chicken in commercial barbecue sauce or prepared breadcrumb mixes.

- For cakes and cookies, use cream (instead of milk) diluted with water, and only use the egg yolk rather than of the whole egg (see A&B Method recipes). Yeast is Neutral and therefore perfect for baking cookies and cakes.

- Eat raw vegetables as frequently as possible. If you need to cook vegetables, then steam them to hold as many vitamins as possible. Whenever you eat acid-building foods, such as cooked meat, cooked fish, sausages and cheese below 50% fat, try to eat them with fresh fruits (but not "A"-bananas, grapes, figs and dates). It tastes good and balances the acid-alkaline in our bodies.

A Tip for Working People

If you bring your lunch to work, be sure to include either fruits from the "B" group or any kind of vegetable salad. You can eat the A&B Method Power Salad (see recipe in cookbook) and "B" fruits with cottage cheese, goat or ewe's milk cheese, feta, mozzarella, or cream cheese, Roquefort, ricotta, or anything from the Neutral group. Many of these same type foods are readily available at salad bars in the local supermarket or deli.

Be careful with ready-mixed salad dressings, especially during the first phase of detoxifying your system. Most of them contain sugar, flour, corn syrup and chemicals. Even so, there are plenty of salad dressings and dips available which are fresh. Check the labels. If you want to play it safe, use vinegar or lemon, olive oil, sea salt and pepper.

Chapter 20

QUESTIONS AND ANSWERS
From A to Z

ALCOHOL *"What about alcohol? Do I have to stop drinking, or can I have an occasional glass of wine or beer?"*

BEER is slightly acid-building, on the boundary of being Neutral—i.e., moderate base-building. You can drink it with any food from Neutral and "A."

DRY WINE is moderately acid-building, and you can drink it with any food from the Neutral and "B" group. CHAMPAGNE and SWEET WINE are also strong acid-builders, but you can drink them with any food from the Neutral or "B" group.

Rye WHISKEY and GIN belong to the Neutral group, despite being strong acid-builders.

(Acid-building alcohol should be avoided if your health doesn't allow it. If you have health problems, you should discuss the amounts with your doctor.)

|BEANS| *"What about beans?"*
Beans are believed to be difficult to digest. But if this were really true, how could this food item be the national dish of so many countries? Until the turn of the last century, beans were the national dish not only in Arabia, but also in Europe, Africa, Asia, and Middle and South America, until our Economic Miracle changed our eating habits forever. However, being the "national dish," means, automatically, that the food must be healthy, must taste good, and must be inexpensive. The truth is that all *fresh beans* as well as peas or lentils, which are all part of the food group "legume" *are base-builders* before drying. (Acid-forming dried beans become alkaline-forming when sprouted. Alkaline-forming dried soybeans, however, increase their alkaline dramatically when sprouted.) Among 500 different types of beans, there are the well-known brown, white, and Garbanzo beans (chickpeas), but also the less-known fava beans. The small and skinless fava beans are the Egyptian national dish (see A&B Cookbook recipe "Ramses Beans") that also includes Garbanzo beans and lentils. This dish is the backbone of the Egyptian farmers' nutrition, and they are probably one of the healthiest people on earth. The Egyptians don't have any problem digesting the beans because they prepare them properly. The Egyptians soak the beans in water for a couple of hours; this prepares them (unknowingly) for a chemical process that makes digestion easier. *Moreover, the Egyptians are eating the Ramses Beans the way they ought to be eaten:* with base-builders, wheat bread and olive oil.

They always eat their dish either with several raw onions (prepared with vinegar, pepper, salt, and cumin, crushing the onions gently with their hand for the sake of the spices) or with only fresh radish, or special salads, such as the Ramses Salad. The Egyptians, like all Arabs, rarely eat kidney beans, white and brown beans, or beans in cans. These beans require an even more complicated preparation process and are, ultimately, difficult to digest. But the main reason for the preference of Arabian connoisseurs is most certainly that fava beans have a particular taste that makes Ramses Beans so delicious.

CANNED FOOD *"What about canned food?"*
Canned fruits and vegetables are not recommended because most of the vitamins are destroyed during the cooking process. Many canned fish products contain water and salt; if you are healthy this is ok from time to time. The same is true for canned meat and sausages. Avoid canned food that contains sugar, corn and flour.

CEREAL AND MILK *"Can I add milk to my cereal?"*
If you are used to adding milk to your cereal (hopefully without sugar), then, instead of milk, use yogurt or cream, plain or diluted with water. It's the same taste—with a different chemistry. This is also valid for baking cakes, cookies and sweets. Replace the milk with cream diluted with water.

CHEESE *"What about cheese? Is it true that I should avoid dairy products?"*

Not at all. Cheese with a fat content above 60% is Neutral and is healthy. It can be eaten with bread (preferably, wheat bread) and anything from "A:, "B", and, of course, Neutral. But cheese with fat content below 50% ("B," right column) is an acid-builder. Limit your amounts of cheese below 50% fat and American processed cheese, pasteurized and processed cheese foods. These "B" cheeses can be eaten with anything from "B" and Neutral but not with bread, pizza, noodles, or anything from "A" (left column.) Try to eat cheese below 50% fat with "B"-fruits from the right side ("B") or Neutral fruits. Eliminate low-fat/fat-free cheese products. Not only don't they taste as good as regular cheese but also they contain unhealthy and/or incompatible acid-building sugar and artificial additives. If you are in the process of losing weight or if your cholesterol is high, restrict not only cheese below 50% fat but also cheese above 60% fat.

CHEWING *"Why is chewing so important?"*

Chew your carbohydrates (such as bread, potatoes, noodles) extremely well to activate the enzyme amylase, for digestion. Carbohydrates ("A," left column) should be chewed, according to the latest research, 25 to 40 times. Saliva is needed for the first step in carbohydrate digestion (and its action) due to the enzyme amylase. If you chew well, your digestive organs have to make less effort. If you don't chew enough, your digestive organs are burdened and stressed.

CHOCOLATE "*Is it true that chocolate makes you fat?*"
No! Yet, white sugar ("A") and brown sugar products are not really recommended. Still, even unhealthy carbohydrates *(gray)* are not as damaging as the "extreme-bad" and "bad" proteins. Therefore, chocolate and sweets ("A") may be eaten moderately with other food from the Neutral and "A" column, but NOT with items from "B." You will find in the cookbook section a number of recipes for cakes, cookies, and other sweets that taste great but are chemically correct.

DIPS and SALAD DRESSING
Although ready-made food is not recommended due to its chemical additives and fillers like sugar, flour, and corn syrup, there are plenty of salad dressings and dips available which are fresh and produced without preservatives. Read the labels. You can find creamy Italian garlic dip, Blue Cheese dips, and others. As long as those dips and salad dressings are used with your A&B salad (with cauliflower, broccoli, spinach, onion, carrots, salad, and any kind of vegetables you like), minor chemicals that might be added won't make a big difference. The most important point is that you get as many fresh vegetables and salads in your system as possible.

DRIED FRUITS "*What about dried fruits?*"
Dried fruits, unsulfured, are great. Dried fruits, sulfured, such as apples and pears, are less recommended but acceptable.

EGGS *"What about eggs?"*
Do not eat (whole) eggs more than three times a week; avoid egg white (albumin)—but *egg yolks are healthy.* The egg yolk is Neutral and the whole egg belongs to "B." Spread wheat bread with mayonnaise and crumble the cooked egg yolk over your bread, or mash the egg yolk and add mayonnaise to a spreading consistence. You will be surprised how delicious it tastes.

FATS *"What about healthy fats?"*
Butter and natural oils such as olive oils, sunflower oils, flaxseed oils, soy oils, and sesame oils, are healthy. A total of 60 to 80 grams of fat for moderately active men and women and teenage girls and boys is a healthy daily allowance. The amount of healthy fats should be individually adjusted to the activity of a person. People with health problems should discuss the amount with their medical doctor. Avoid industrialized oils.

FAT-FREE/LOW-FAT PRODUCTS *"Will eating fat-free or low-fat products help me to lose weight?"*
Not at all. If this were the case, it would be easy to lose weight because you would just need to avoid eating fat. Many people consume these products without being able to correct their weight problems. Let's face it: how much fat can you eat over the course of a day in order to reach a total of 60 to 80 grams, which is all right for a healthy and moderately active person? Moreover, low-fat and fat-free products contain sugar and artificial additives, which interfere with your body's chemistry, thus metabolism. This is not only very unhealthy, but above all, it interferes with the A&B principles.

Therefore, eliminate low-fat and fat-free products completely from your menu. Replace them with healthy oils and their vital minerals and vitamins, such as vitamin E. *Instead* of eating low-fat or fat-free products, *eat,* for example, cauliflower. It is high in pantothenic acid and *it demolishes fat.* It plays a central role in the biochemical reactions within the body.

FISH (COOKED) *"What about cooked fish?"*
Cooked fish is an acid-builder. Try to eat the fish with "B"- or Neutral fruits, vegetables, and salads. But check with the A&B Chart. You will find that there are smoked herring, smoked mackerel, smoked trout, smoked salmon, and marinated white herring in the Neutral group, which taste great but are chemically different. Fish is better for us than cooked meat.

HONEY *"Is honey healthy?"*
Yes! Pure natural honey (cold rinsed) is highly recommended. Other honey is less recommended but acceptable. Honey ("A") may be eaten with any other food from "A" and Neutral, but not with foods from the "B" group (right column).

MARGARINE *"Is margarine better than butter?"*
Although it is a vegetable product, and Neutral, the use of commercial margarine is not recommended. The heating process breaks hydrogen bonds, creating a product that causes rancidity and hardening in the tissues. Butter (a moderate base-builder) is much more digestible than margarine and is therefore recommended.

MAYONNAISE *"Is it true that mayonnaise makes me fat?"* Not at all! Mayonnaise belongs to the Neutral group (middle column) and may be eaten like all fats and oils with "A," "B," and/or Neutral.

MEAT (COOKED) *"What about cooked meat?"*
Meat is a strong acid-builder. You should eat it only from time to time. However, if you eat cooked/fried meat, then try to eat it with vegetables, salads, and fruits. However, there are Neutral meat products such as bacon, smoked ham, rolled ham, cured meat, and dried meat, which taste great, and their chemistry fits the body chemistry.

MILK *"Will I get diarrhea from drinking milk!"*
You might go through the so-called Healing Crisis, while the body works hard to get rid of the poison. You might have diarrhea, headache, and shooting pains. The reaction differs, due to age or the progress of the disease. After approximately one week on the A&B Method, the body begins to better tolerate the milk.

MILK and COFFEE *"What about milk in my coffee?"*
If you eat wheat bread with honey and some cottage cheese and at the same time you drink your coffee, use cream or cream diluted with water instead of milk for the coffee. But if you eat food from the "B" or Neutral groups you can drink your coffee with regular milk.

READY-MADE FOOD *"What about ready-made food?"*
Limit, preferably eliminate, ready-made foods because of artificial additives, sugar, corn syrup, corn starch, fructose, bread crumbs, bleached flours, acetic acid, cooked tomatoes, and many chemicals.

SALAD DRESSINGS See Dips.

SWEETENING *"How should I sweeten foods, coffee and tea?"*
Sweeten with sugar substitute, fresh fruits, or pure honey (cold rinsed). Other honey is less recommended but acceptable. Since honey is in the "A" group (left column) it may be eaten with other foods from "A" and Neutrals but should not be added to foods from the "B" group (right column).

SOY PRODUCTS *"What about soy products?"*
Before processing, soybeans are strong base-builders. However, soy flour (made of soy beans), soy imitations, and soy ready-mixtures turn into moderate acid-builders (*white* on the A&B Chart) after processing and belong to the Neutral group.

SOY SPROUTS/SOY SAUCE
Soy sprouts and soy oil are Neutral (middle column) and base-builders (*yellow* on the A&B Chart). They are indeed healthy. This is also valid for soy sauce.

TOFU "*Is it true that tofu has the power to cure cancer?*"

Tofu (made from soy beans) is a high-grade protein food item (but Neutral, like all leguminous plant foods, such as beans, lentils, and peas: *white* on the A&B Chart). Please read Chapter 9.

WEIGHT "*Do I need to weigh myself every day?*"

You don't need to weigh yourself every day. Just let it go. There are phases during the healing crisis when you won't see any change on the scale. Since your body is getting rid of its poison, your weight regulates itself. If you are overweight, you will lose weight. If you are underweight, you will gain weight. At the beginning, we suggest you stick with the A&B principles and not interrupt the important work of the body's chemistry until you have reached your goal. You can weigh yourself every week.

WRONG EATING "*What if I ate wrong?*"

If you already detoxified your body and your acid-alkaline balance is in good shape (and you lost the weight as you wanted) it might happen that you can't resist "eating wrong." For example, you eat a complete meal in a fast food restaurant, such as hamburger on a roll and french fries with a milkshake (which is A&B at the same time). Don't worry. You just need to go back to the A&B and you will soon be back on track towards health. It takes a few days to gain weight. A detoxified body can easily deal with mistakes for a while.

In case you start to feel bad, immediately eat some raw vegetables, salads, and/or fruits to increase your alkaline levels. The best vegetables to use for this purpose are (besides Neutral and "B"-fruits) raw vegetables and salads, such as root vegetables, carrots (add a few drops of oil to make it easier for your body to utilize the valuable vitamin A), turnips, beets, and all sorts of top vegetables, such as spinach, sprouts, beet tops, chard, celery, onion tops, watercress, broccoli, cauliflower, or any green vegetable that contains juice. These vitamins and minerals will enable your metabolism to do its job. Soon you will feel better.

ZERO CALORIE COUNTING *"Should I count calories?"*
No! The idea of "calories" stems from the time when the steam engine was born: put in coal and out comes energy. At that time people believed that it must be the same with food. The idea is simplistic and limited in scope: we are not steamboats, which work with steam engines that must be fueled—we are a BioChemical Machine, which works upon the laws of our body's own chemistry.

PART IX

Cookbook

The cookbook has been created not only with a view toward good health, but for all lifestyles. There are recipes for LEVEL ONE and LEVEL TWO. You should choose the dishes according to the level you are using.

Special recognition is awarded to
Sylvia Bennett
for her development of the following recipes, aligned to chemical compatibility of the body's biochemistry.

BREAKFAST "A"

Milk & Apples

The best breakfast is indeed milk (or yogurt) with apples, because it is first of all detoxifying, but also you will be not hungry for hours to come. You will feel as if you had eaten a complete traditional breakfast. Apples are high in fiber; a medium apple contains 9–10 grams of fiber, a good portion of the 20–35 grams you need every day. One glass of milk (250 ml) contains 8 grams of fat, which is a fragment of the 60–80 grams of fat that are healthy for a moderately active person. But remember: apples and milk are "B" and should not be used in combination with an "A" breakfast. However, if you cannot instantly change your eating habits, then you will find, in the following, some ideas for a healthy "traditional" breakfast.

Classic Cereal Breakfast

1. In a large bowl, add cereal (if possible, without sugar).
2. Add
   a) Natural whole milk yogurt,
   b) Cream (diluted with water), or
   c) Sour cream.
3. Combine the cereal to taste: with bananas, blueberries, raisins, dates, dried figs, honey, and/or all kinds of nuts (including peanuts, because they belong to "A").

OPTIONAL: Bagel with cream cheese

OPTIONAL: Wheat bread/rye (toast) with butter and honey or jam/jelly/marmalade. If you don't like it so sweet, then choose a wheat bread/rye bread (toast) with butter or mayonnaise and slices of tomatoes, onions (or cucumber), and salt; or fresh bread with butter, cottage cheese, and/or cream cheese, Camembert, goat's milk cheese, ewe's milk cheese, egg yolk (only), chives, and salt.

Classic Muesli

1 tablespoon cottage cheese (or ricotta cheese)
1 banana
2 tablespoons nuts, grated
2 tablespoons raisins (or dates)
1 tablespoon wheat bran
1 tablespoon fresh flaxseed, crushed
3 tablespoons wheat germ (*)

> In a medium bowl, combine cottage cheese/ricotta and banana. Mix well. Add remaining ingredients.

(*) Wheat germ: Much too ugly of a name for a great and good tasting product which is full of vitamins, especially vitamin E; 3 tablespoons a day will do "miracles" for your health.

Fruit Muesli

Banana (and/or fresh or dried figs, dried apples,
    dried plums, dried dates, raisins)
2 tablespoons flaxseeds, crushed
2 tablespoons flaxseed oil
6 tablespoons buttermilk
1 tablespoon honey
Walnuts, grated
1 1/2 cups cottage cheese, or ricotta
1 tablespoon honey

1. In a medium bowl, combine fruit with flaxseeds and 4 tablespoons buttermilk.
2. In medium bowl, combine cottage cheese (or ricotta) with 2 tablespoons buttermilk, honey, and flaxseed oil. Spread mixture over muesli; top with walnuts.

Fresh-Grain Muesli

1–3 figs (or dates)
1/2 cup raisins, soaked in water for 5 hours
1/2 cup grain, oat or wheat flakes
1 cup cream
1 banana, mashed (or 1 cup blueberries)

1. In a medium bowl with water, soak raisins for 5 hours.
2. Drain raisins and combine all ingredients.

Fresh Herb-Grain Breakfast

1 cup cottage cheese (or ricotta)
4 tablespoons wheat germ
2 tablespoons sunflower oil
4 tablespoons sour cream
1/4 cup chives
1/8 cup chervil
1 pinch of herb-salt (OPTIONAL: sea salt)

In a medium bowl, combine ingredients. Serve with wheat bread.

LUNCH
and
DINNER
"A"

PIZZA "A"

In the following you will find two BASIC RECIPES you need for
every type of pizza:

A&B PIZZA DOUGH and A&B PIZZA SAUCE.

a) A&B Pizza Sauce replaces the common but chemically incompatible tomato sauce.
b) A&B Pizza Dough should be made from whole wheat flour or frozen wheat bread dough (thawed as package directs).

A&B PIZZA DOUGH
Basic Recipe

2 cups whole wheat flour
1 tablespoon yeast
1 1/2 cups water
2 tablespoons olive oil
1 tablespoon butter
1 teaspoon sea salt

1. In a medium mixing bowl combine flour, yeast, oil, salt, and water. Stir mixture together with your hands until dough is firm but moist (if necessary, add more water, 1 tablespoon at time). Let dough rest for 1 hour.
2. Knead dough again with your hands. Cover and let rise in a warm place (20 minutes).
3. Preheat oven to 350°F. Sprinkle whole wheat flour over greased baking sheet.
4. Using a rolling pin, roll out dough on baking sheet. Arrange toppings.

A&B PIZZA SAUCE
Basic Recipe

1 cup ricotta cheese
3 cloves garlic
1/2 cup heavy cream
1 teaspoon oregano
1 teaspoon dried parsley
1 teaspoon basil
1 tablespoon olive oil

In a food processor, combine cheese, garlic, cream, oregano, parsley, and basil. Process until a paste forms. Slowly add oil; set aside until A&B Pizza Dough is ready.

Pizza Romana

A&B Pizza Dough and A&B Pizza Sauce (basic recipe)
1 large onion, sliced
1 large green pepper, sliced
1/2 pound mushrooms, sliced
2 cloves garlic, grated
1/2 pound leeks, chopped
1/2 pound ewe's milk cheese
1 cup sour cream
1 tablespoon fresh basil, chopped (or 1 teaspoon dried)
Dried oregano to taste
1/2 pound olives
3 cups mozzarella, shredded

1. Prepare Pizza Dough.
2. Prepare Pizza Sauce.
3. In a small saucepan, steam onions until tender but not brown. Add chopped leeks, 1 cup ewe's milk cheese, basil, and sour cream.
4. Spread mixture evenly over dough. Cut remaining ewe's milk cheese in quarters. Top pizza with olives, pepper, onions, mushrooms, and ewe's milk cheese. Sprinkle mozzarella and oregano evenly over the pizza. Bake at 350°F on lowest shelf (or the floor of a gas oven) until crust is firm and nicely brown at edges, 20–25 minutes. Cut into serving pieces and serve warm.

Mozzarella Pizza

A&B Pizza Dough and A&B Pizza Sauce (basic recipe)
3 cups mozzarella cheese (about 12 ounces), shredded
2 tablespoons pine nuts

1. Prepare Pizza Dough.
2. Prepare Pizza Sauce.
3. Spread Pizza Sauce evenly over dough. Top with mozzarella and pine nuts. Place baking sheet on lowest shelf in oven (or the floor of a gas oven). Bake at 350°F until crust is firm and nicely brown, 15 to 20 minutes. Serve warm.

Pizza Via Veneto

A&B Pizza Dough and A&B Pizza Sauce (basic recipe)
1 jar/can artichoke hearts
2 medium onions, sliced
1/4 cup vegetable or olive oil
3 cups mozzarella, shredded
1 tablespoon oregano, chopped fresh (or 1 teaspoon dried)
2 tablespoons olive oil

1. Prepare Pizza Dough.
2. Prepare Pizza Sauce.
3. In a large frying pan, cook onions in oil, stirring occasionally, until tender. Add artichokes, cheese, and oregano; set aside.
4. Spread Pizza Sauce evenly over dough. Top with artichoke hearts, mozzarella, and oregano. Drizzle remaining oil over pizza and bake at 350°F on lowest shelf (or the floor of a gas oven) until crust is firm and nicely brown at edges, 15–20 minutes. Serve warm.

Pizza Napoli

A&B Pizza Dough and A&B Pizza Sauce (basic recipe)
1 1/2 cups feta cheese, shredded
Olives (any kind, quantity to taste)
3 cups mozzarella, shredded

1. Prepare Pizza Dough.
2. Prepare Pizza Sauce.
3. Spread Pizza Sauce evenly over dough. Top with feta and olives. Sprinkle mozzarella evenly over the pizza. Place baking sheet on lowest shelf in oven and bake until crust is firm and nicely brown, 15–20 minutes. Serve warm.

Pizza Venetian

A&B Pizza Dough and A&B Pizza Sauce (basic recipe)
1 large eggplant
2 cups mozzarella, shredded
4 cloves garlic, chopped or crushed
1 large onion, chopped (for eggplants)
1 large onion, sliced into rings (for pizza)
1 green pepper, sliced
1 teaspoon oregano
1 teaspoon basil
1 teaspoon parsley
1/2 cup olive oil

1. Cut eggplant into 3/4-inch quarters. Put eggplant in a strainer. Sprinkle sufficient salt over eggplant. Let stand until fluid is removed, 45 minutes. In a large saucepan, cook eggplant in hot oil until brown. Add onions and garlic, turning, until eggplant is nicely brown; set aside.
2. Prepare Pizza Dough.
3. Prepare Pizza Sauce.
4. Spread Pizza Sauce over dough. Top with pieces of eggplant. Sprinkle oregano, parsley, and basil. Top with mozzarella and onion rings. Place baking sheet on lowest shelf in oven (or the floor of a gas oven) and bake at 350°F until crust is firm and nicely brown, 15–20 minutes. Serve warm.

Pizza Milanese

A&B Pizza Dough and A&B Pizza Sauce (basic recipe)
1/2 pound mushrooms, sliced
2 large leeks, sliced
1 large onion, sliced into rings
1–2 pepper, sliced into rings
Olives (any kind, quantity to taste)
Sea salt

1. Prepare Pizza Dough and Pizza Sauce.
2. Spread sauce evenly over dough. Top with mushrooms, leeks, onion rings, pepper rings, and olives. Place baking sheet on lowest shelf in oven (or the floor of a gas oven) and bake at 350°F until crust is firm and nicely brown, 15–20 minutes. Serve warm.

Pizza A&B Four Seasons

A&B Pizza Dough and A&B Pizza Sauce (basic recipe)
Broccoli, quantity to taste
Cauliflower, quantity to taste
Mushrooms, quantity to taste
1/2 eggplant
1 large onion, sliced into rings
Olives (quantity to taste)
3 cups mozzarella, shredded

1. Cut eggplant into 3/4-inch quarters. Put eggplant in a strainer. Sprinkle sufficient salt over eggplant. Let stand until fluid is removed, 45 minutes. In a large saucepan, cook eggplant in hot oil until brown. Add onions and garlic, turning, until eggplant is nicely brown; set aside.
2. Prepare Pizza Dough.
3. Prepare Pizza Sauce.
4. Spread Pizza Sauce evenly over dough. Top with broccoli, cauliflower, mushrooms, eggplants, onions, olives. Sprinkle mozzarella evenly over the pizza. Place baking sheet on lowest shelf in oven (or the floor of a gas oven) and bake at 350°F until crust is firm and nicely brown, 15–20 minutes. Serve warm.

PASTA "A"

It would be in your best interest to buy pasta made from whole wheat flour. (However, you can eat white flour from time to time, especially in restaurants, if health reasons are not your main concern.) Pasta should be served with mixed salads and/or may be eaten with bananas, grapes, fresh figs, fresh dates, dried apples, dried plums, dried figs, dried dates, raisins, and all kind of nuts (including peanuts). Beer, whiskey, rye and gin are compatible.

THE A&B WHITE SAUCE IS A BASIC SAUCE
THAT CAN BE USED FOR EVERY PASTA DISH.

A&B WHITE SAUCE
Basic Recipe

6 tablespoons butter
4 tablespoons wheat flour
1 cup heavy cream (diluted with 2 cups water)
Pinch of sea salt and freshly ground pepper
Pinch of grated nutmeg, optional

In a saucepan, melt butter over low heat. Slowly add flour as butter melts; stir until smooth. Pour in cream, stirring constantly for 15 minutes or until smooth and velvety. Increase heat and stir until sauce comes to a boil. Low simmer for 10 minutes more, stirring occasionally. Add salt, pepper, and nutmeg to taste. Whisk again until the sauce is smooth.

Rigatoni with Broccoli and A&B White Sauce (OPTIONAL: Fusilli)

4 servings

1 pound rigatoni or fusilli
1 bunch fresh broccoli, washed and stems cut off
1/2 cup chopped olives, black and green
1/2 pound fatty bacon, chopped
3 cloves garlic, minced or pressed
1/4 cup dry white wine
7-oz can chicken broth (or 1 cup bouillon)
2 tablespoons butter
1/2 cup fresh Italian parsley, chopped
1 tablespoon basil
1/2 cup olive oil
1 cup A&B White Sauce

1. Prepare A&B White Sauce; set aside.
2. In a saucepan, lightly brown oil, garlic, and bacon for 10 minutes. Add wine and let simmer over medium heat for 5 minutes. Add broken-up broccoli, salt, and pepper to taste; let cook for 10 minutes. Add chicken broth and 1 cup A&B White Sauce; simmer for 5 minutes. Add olives, basil, parsley, and butter; simmer another 3 minutes.
3. While sauce is simmering, cook pasta in boiling salted water until tender but firm. Remove from heat and drain. Place in warm bowl and mix with broccoli sauce. Serve immediately.

Rigatoni à la Gondola   4 servings

1 pound rigatoni
5 pieces dried mushrooms
1 cup heavy cream
1/2 cup feta cheese, shredded
Fresh oregano to taste
Fresh basil to taste
3 cloves garlic, crushed through a press
1/4 cup olive oil
Olives, chopped (quantity to taste)

1. In a food processor, crush mushrooms; set aside.
2. In a frying pan, cook olive oil; add garlic, oregano, basil, and heavy cream (2 minutes.) Add feta cheese; set aside.
3. In a large saucepan, cook rigatoni in boiling salted water until tender but firm. Remove from heat and drain. Pour mixture over rigatoni. Mix well. Sprinkle crushed mushrooms together with chopped olives over rigatoni.

Spaghetti à la Toscana   4 servings

1/2 pound spaghetti
4 onions, chopped
2 large cloves garlic, crushed through a press
1 1/2 pounds mushrooms, sliced
2 tablespoons butter
1/2 pound grated fresh cheese (above 60% fat)
1 cup heavy cream
1 teaspoon fresh basil, chopped
1 pinch sea salt
1 pinch pepper
1 teaspoon basil
1 teaspoon oregano

1. In a medium saucepan, cook onions and mushrooms in butter until softened but not brown. Add garlic, salt, and pepper to taste. Add fresh cheese. Cook until melted. Add cream. Mix well; set aside.
2. In a large saucepan, cook pasta in boiling salted water until tender but firm. Remove from heat and drain. Sprinkle mixture over spaghetti. Drizzle fresh basil and oregano to taste.

Fettucine Alfredo   4 servings

1 pound fettucine
8 tablespoons butter, softened
1/4 cup heavy cream
1 cup grated mozzarella cheese
Freshly ground pepper

1. Cook pasta in boiling salted water until tender but firm. Remove from heat and drain.
2. Place fettucine in a warm bowl or on a serving platter. Add butter, cream, and half the mozzarella cheese. Toss fettucine noodles gently until they are evenly coated. Serve immediately, topped with pepper and remaining mozzarella cheese.

Spaghetti à la Bell Paese   4 servings

1/2 pound spaghetti
2 large tomatoes
1 bundle fresh basil
Parsley to taste
3 sticks celery
4 cloves garlic, crushed through a press
2 fresh green onions
1/2 tablespoon fresh oregano
Olive oil
Sea salt to taste
Pepper to taste
Seasoning to taste

1. Cut all vegetables in very small pieces (don't cook). Add lemon and olive oil. Mix well.
2. In a large saucepan, cook spaghetti in boiling salted water until tender but firm. Remove from heat and drain. Spread mixture over spaghetti.

Pasta di Paesano   4 servings

1/2 pound elbow noodles
Feta cheese (quantity to taste)
1 cup heavy cream
4 cloves garlic, crushed through a press
Fresh mint (quantity to taste), chopped
Fresh spinach (quantity to taste), chopped
Olive oil

1. Combine (uncooked) spinach, mint, feta cheese, cream, olive oil, and garlic; set aside.
2. In a saucepan, cook noodles in boiling salted water until tender but firm. Remove from heat and drain. Add mixture to noodles. Mix well.

Spaghetti with Four Cheeses   4 servings

1 pound spaghetti
2 oz feta cheese
2 oz cream Gouda cheese
2 oz Gorgonzola (Italian soft blue cheese)
2 oz cottage cheese
1/4 cup butter
Sea salt to taste

1. Dice all cheese, except cottage cheese, into 1/4-inch cubes; place in a bowl; set aside.
2. Cook pasta in boiling salted water until tender but firm. Remove from heat and drain. Place spaghetti back into the same pot and add butter and diced cheese.
3. Simmer over medium heat until cheese is melted. Remove from heat and place in warm bowl. Sprinkle with cottage cheese and serve immediately.

Pasta à la Chinoise   4 servings

1/2 pound spaghetti
4 carrots, sliced
1 1/2 pounds mushrooms, sliced
4 scallions, sliced
2 stalks celery, sliced
Onion, sliced into rings
2 large cloves garlic, crushed through a press or chopped
Butter to taste (or olive oil)
Soy sauce to taste
Cayenne pepper to taste
Ginger to taste
Sea salt to taste
Pepper to taste

1. In a large saucepan or wok, cook onions until golden brown. Gradually add carrots, mushrooms, celery, scallions, garlic, soy sauce, cayenne pepper, ginger, salt and pepper in butter or olive oil until brown; set aside.
2. In a saucepan, cook pasta in boiling salted water until tender but firm. Remove from heat and drain.
3. Add spaghetti to mixture. Mix well.

Macaroni and Cheese   4 servings

1/2 pound macaroni
3 cups mozzarella, shredded
4–5 cloves garlic, crushed through a press
1 teaspoon oregano
1 teaspoon thyme

1. In a large saucepan, cook macaroni in boiling salted water until tender but firm. Remove from heat and drain.
2. Combine oregano, thyme, and garlic. Sprinkle mixture over macaroni. Sprinkle mozzarella evenly over the macaroni.
3. Preheat oven to 300°F. Place macaroni in a greased baking dish. Bake until macaroni is nicely brown and crisp, about 20 minutes.

Pasta Parisian   4 servings

1/2 pound rigatoni (or any other type of pasta)
1 large eggplant
1 cup ricotta cheese (or cottage cheese)
1/2 cup heavy cream (diluted with little water)
1/2 cup olive oil
2 large cloves garlic, crushed through a press
2 carrots, cut into thin strips
2 celery stalks, cut into thin strips
4 onions, chopped
Soy sauce to taste
1 teaspoon oregano
1 teaspoon basil
Cayenne pepper to taste

1. Cut eggplant into 3/4-inch cubes. Put eggplant in a strainer. Sprinkle sufficient salt over eggplant. Let stand until fluid is removed, 45 minutes.
2. In a saucepan, cook pasta in boiling salted water until tender but firm. Remove from heat and drain.
3. In a deep frying pan or wok, cook onions, and garlic in hot oil until brown. Add eggplant. Spice with soy sauce, oregano, basil, and cayenne pepper. Reduce heat; cook, stirring occasionally, at least 1/2 hour. Add ricotta (or cottage) cheese as well as 1/2 cup heavy cream. Add mixture to rigatoni. Mix well.

Angel's Hair (Capelli d'Angelo)   4 servings
with Mushrooms

1 pound capelli d'angelo
20 whole button mushrooms, cleaned
1/2 pound butter
Freshly ground pepper
4 tablespoons grated mozzarella

Cook pasta in boiling salted water for 1 minute until tender but firm. Sauté mushrooms in butter for 10 minutes or until soft. Add pepper. In a large, warm bowl, place half mushroom mixture; add capelli d'angelo and toss gently. Sprinkle in mozzarella cheese and toss again. Serve warm with mushrooms and butter sauce spooned over.

Angel's Hair Soufflé (Capelli d'Angelo)   4 servings

1/2 pound capelli d'angelo
4 egg yolks, separated
1/2 cup grated mozzarella
1 cup A&B White Sauce

1. Prepare A&B White Sauce; set aside.
2. Cook pasta in boiling salted water for 1 minute or until tender but firm. Remove from heat and drain. In a mixing bowl, combine egg yolks and mozzarella cheese. Mix until stiff.
3. Mix in capelli d'angelo and blend thoroughly.
4. Pour mixture into a buttered soufflé dish. Bake at 450°F, or until soufflé puffs up. Serve immediately with A&B White Sauce.

Pasta "Decamerone"   4 servings

1/2 pound rigatoni (or any other type of pasta)
1 1/2 pounds mushrooms, sliced
1 can green peas
2 tablespoons butter
2 cups heavy cream
1 cup cream cheese
4 onions, chopped
2 large cloves garlic, crushed through a press

1. In a medium saucepan, cook onions and mushrooms in butter until softened but not brown. Add peas (without fluid), garlic, salt, and pepper to taste. Add heavy cream and cream cheese. Mix well; set aside.
2. In a large saucepan, cook pasta in boiling salted water until tender but firm. Remove from heat and drain. Sprinkle mixture over pasta. Mix well.

Rigatoni with Garlic   4 servings

1 pound rigatoni
5 tablespoons olive oil
2 cloves garlic, minced or pressed
Pinch of sea salt
Pinch of freshly ground pepper
3 sprigs rosemary

Cook pasta in boiling salted water until tender but firm. While pasta is cooking, fry garlic, rosemary, salt, and pepper in oil until garlic is golden brown. Add 2 tablespoons of the water in which the rigatoni is cooking; stir. Remove rosemary from oil mixture. When rigatoni is cooked, remove from heat and drain. Place in a warm bowl; mix with the flavored oil and serve immediately.

Trenette with Pesto   4 servings

1 pound trenette
4 garlic cloves, crushed
2 cups fresh basil leaves, crushed
Sea salt to taste
1 teaspoon olive oil
1 cup grated mozzarella cheese
1/2 cup pine nuts

1. Crush basil leaves with a mortar and pestle, gradually adding salt and garlic cloves. When all the garlic and basil is thoroughly crushed, start to add mozzarella cheese. Continue to grind until all the ingredients form a fairly thick consistency. Dilute with olive oil. Now the pesto sauce is ready.
2. Cook pasta in boiling salted water until tender but firm. Remove from heat and drain. Place trenette in a warm bowl and add pesto sauce; mix thoroughly until all noodles are evenly coated.

VARIETY "A"

Mushroom Soufflé   4 servings

1 1/2 cups whole rye flour or 1/2 cup whole wheat flour
1/2 pound butter
1/2 cup water
1 pound mushrooms, sliced
1 small onion, chopped
1 egg yolk
1 cup heavy cream
Sea salt to taste
Pepper to taste

1. In a medium mixing bowl, combine whole rye flour or whole wheat flour, butter, sea salt, and 1/2 cup water. Stir mixture together with your hands.
2. Preheat oven to 350°F. Brush soufflé pan with butter before placing 2/3 of the dough on baking sheet. Reserve 1/3 of the dough; set aside.
3. In a small saucepan, fry chopped onions. Add mushrooms, egg yolks, heavy cream, and spices. Let cook 10 minutes.
4. Place mixture on dough. Cover soufflé with remaining dough. Bake until brown and crispy.

POTATOES "A"

The potato is full of vitamin C, calcium, and phosphorus, but the richest concentration of minerals is directly under the skin. Therefore, cook potatoes in their jackets (unpeeled in the vegetable steamer), instead of peeling them before cooking.

Austrian Baked Potatoes "Arnold"   4 servings

Potatoes, quantity to taste
Butter (1 tablespoon for each potato)
Sour cream, OR ready-to-buy fresh creamy Italian garlic dip,
          OR fresh sour cream dip without preservatives
Aluminum wrap
Parsley and chives
Sea salt
Pepper

1.   With a sharp knife, make a 1-inch cut across each potato. Season potatoes with salt and pepper to taste. Top each potato with a tablespoon of butter. Wrap each potato in aluminum wrap.
2.   Preheat oven to 400°F. Place potatoes on baking sheet. Bake until tender, approximately 30 minutes.
3.   In a bowl, combine sour cream with parsley and chives to taste. Serve warm (in its aluminum wrap).

Stove-Top Potato Casserole   4 servings

4 large potatoes, steamed and 1/4-inch sliced
4 zucchinis, 1/4-inch sliced
1 large onion, sliced
4 egg yolks
1/2 cup mozzarella, shredded
Herbs to taste
Dried parsley to taste
4 tablespoons butter or oil

1. In a vegetable steamer, place potatoes over boiling water, 20 minutes. Add zucchini. Cook until tender. Place potatoes in a large bowl. Let stand until potatoes are cool enough to handle. Peel and slice potatoes.
2. In a small bowl, whisk egg yolks. Add mozzarella. Mix well; set aside.
3. In a medium saucepan, cook onions in butter (or olive oil) until golden brown. Add potatoes and zucchini. Sprinkle egg mixture over potatoes and vegetables. Cook for another 3 minutes. Reduce heat. Cover saucepan. Let stand 15 minutes. Sprinkle herbs over casserole.

Potato Salad Bavaria   4 servings

4 large or 6 small potatoes, (any type)
1 onion, sliced
1/2 bunch parsley, chopped
Vinegar to taste
Olive oil to taste
Sca salt to taste
Pepper to taste

1. In a vegetable steamer, place potatoes over boiling water, 20 minutes. Cook until almost tender. Remove from heat. Place potatoes in a large bowl. Let stand until potatoes are cool enough to handle. Peel potatoes.
2. Cut potatoes into 1/2-inch quarters. Add oil, vinegar, salt, and pepper to taste. Mix well.

Potato Salad d'Alsace   4 servings

6 new potatoes, unpeeled
Beef salami, dice into cubes (OPTIONAL: smoked fish), quantity to taste
1 fresh cucumber, sliced
1 large tomato, sliced in cubes
2 large pickles (sour or sweet dill), chopped into very thin slices
1/2 bunch chives, chopped
Scallions to taste, chopped
1 onion, chopped
Mayonnaise and/or chunky Blue Cheese dressing to taste
Olive or any other natural oil to taste
Vinegar to taste
Sea salt, pepper and celery salt to taste

1. In a vegetable steamer, place potatoes over boiling water for 20–30 minutes. Cook until tender. Remove from heat. Place potatoes in a large bowl. Let stand until potatoes are cool enough to handle. Peel potatoes. Cut potatoes into 1/2-inch cubes.
2. Add oil, vinegar, vegetables, pickled cucumbers, salami (or fish), and mayonnaise to potatoes. Mix well.

Potato Salad Vienna   4 servings

4 large or 6 small potatoes, unpeeled
1 can peas
4 carrots, chopped
1/2 bundle parsley, chopped
Mayonnaise to taste
Oil to taste
Vinegar to taste
Sea salt to taste
Pepper to taste
Garlic powder to taste

1. In a vegetable steamer, place potatoes over boiling water for 20–30 minutes. Cook until tender. Remove from heat.
2. Place potatoes in a large bowl. Let stand until potatoes are cool enough to handle. Peel potatoes. Cut potatoes into 1/2-inch cubes.
3. Add oil, vinegar, carrots, parsley, peas (drained), mayonnaise, salt, pepper, and garlic powder to potatoes. Mix well.

Hungarian Potato Salad with Creamy Dressing

4 servings

6 new potatoes, unpeeled
2 tablespoons butter
1 cup red cabbage, shredded
1–2 tablespoons mayonnaise
1/4 cup olive oil
1 large garlic clove, crushed through a press
1/2 tablespoon sea salt
1/4 teaspoon Hungarian or other paprika
1 tablespoon vinegar
1/2 teaspoon dried thyme
Fresh ground black pepper to taste

1. In a vegetable steamer, place potatoes over boiling water for 20 minutes. Cook until tender. Remove from heat. Place potatoes in a large bowl. Let stand until potatoes are cool enough to handle. Peel potatoes. Cut potatoes into 1/2-inch cubes.
2. In a small saucepan, melt butter. Pour butter over potatoes; add sea salt and paprika and mix well. Add cabbage; set aside.
3. Combine oil, vinegar, salt, garlic, celery salt, herbs, and mayonnaise. Blend well until dressing forms a paste. Pour dressing over potato salad.

Austrian Potato "Pancake"   4 servings

2 medium baking potatoes
1/2 small onion, chopped
1 tablespoon whole wheat flour
1/4 teaspoon baking powder
1/2 cup olive oil
1/2 cup sour cream
2 egg yolks
1 tablespoon minced fresh marjoram (or 1 teaspoon dried)
1/4 teaspoon sea salt
1/8 teaspoon freshly ground pepper

1. In a food processor, grate potatoes, flour, baking powder, and onion. Mix well.
2. Combine marjoram, egg yolks, salt, and pepper. Beat until well blended.
3. In a large frying pan, cook 2 tablespoons oil over medium heat. Drop small portions of potato mix into hot oil and flatten with back of a spoon. Cook, turning once, until golden brown on both sides, about 5 minutes. Drain on paper towels. Top each pancake with sour cream.

New Potatoes Marseilles   4 servings

5 new potatoes, unpeeled
2–3 tablespoons butter, melted
1/4 cup fresh parsley, chopped
sea salt
Pepper

1. In a vegetable steamer, place potatoes over boiling water for 20 minutes. Cook until tender.
2. Remove from heat. Place potatoes in a large bowl. Let stand until potatoes are cool enough to handle. Peel potatoes.
3. Cut potatoes into 1/4-inch slices. Place on baking sheet and brush evenly with butter. Sprinkle with seasoning and place as close as possible to heat of broiler until crusty and golden, for 10 minutes. Sprinkle parsley over potatoes.

Potato Salzburg with Sour Cream   4 servings

10 small new potatoes, unpeeled
1/2 cup sour cream
1/2 bunch chives, minced

1. Preheat oven to 400°F. Arrange potatoes on a baking sheet. Bake potatoes until tender, about 40 minutes. Place potatoes in a large bowl. Let stand until potatoes are cool enough to handle.
2. Peel potatoes. Halve potatoes. Cut a thin slice from the rounded bottom of each potato half so it will stand upright. Using a small spoon, scoop out center from each potato half, leaving a shell about 1/4 inch thick. Using a small spoon, fill each potato cavity with 2 teaspoons sour cream. Cook until heated through, about 10 minutes. Garnish with chives.

Sweet Potato Bites   4 servings

1 pound sweet potatoes (approximately 2-inch diameter)
2 tablespoons olive oil
1/3 cup sour cream

1. Preheat oven to 400°F.
2. Scrub potatoes and trim ends. Cut into 1/4-inch rounds.
3. Brush a baking dish with oil. Arrange sweet potato slices in a single layer; brush tops with remaining oil. Bake 15 minutes or until slices are golden brown on the bottom. Turn slices over. Cook until both sides are nicely brown, 10 minutes.
4. Top with sour cream.

RICE "A"

In the following you will find the BASIC RECIPE for cooking rice. The A&B White Sauce can be used for almost every rice dish.

RICE   2 servings

1 cup natural (brown) rice
1 1/2 tablespoons butter
4 tablespoons olive oil
4 cups chicken broth (or 4 bouillon cubes, dissolved in 4 cups water)

In a medium saucepan, melt butter over medium-low heat. Add rice and cook, stirring, 2–3 minutes. Add 2 cups of broth (or bouillon). Cook rice, stirring, 5–6 minutes. Add 1 more cup broth. Cook until fluid is almost absorbed, 4–5 minutes. Gradually, add remaining broth. Cook, continuously stirring, until rice is tender but firm, about 10–15 minutes. Remove from heat. Let cool.

OPTIONAL:

1. Bring 2 1/2 cups water to boil. Add some sea salt and about 1 teaspoon olive oil or butter, if desired.
2. Add 1 cup rice; stir until thoroughly blended with water. Reduce heat. Cover. Simmer about 20 minutes. Turn off heat. Fluff rice with fork.

A&B WHITE SAUCE

6 tablespoons butter
4 tablespoons whole wheat flour
1 cup heavy cream (diluted with 2 cups water)
Pinch of sea salt and freshly ground pepper
Pinch of grated nutmeg, optional

In a saucepan, melt butter over low heat. Slowly pour in flour as butter melts; stir until smooth. Pour in cream, stirring constantly for 15 minutes or until smooth and velvety. Increase heat and stir until sauce comes to a boil. Simmer for 10 minutes more, stirring occasionally. Add salt, pepper, and nutmeg to taste. Whisk again until the sauce is smooth.

Crispy Rice Balls St. Tropez   4 servings

1 cup brown rice
1 1/2 tablespoons butter
1/4 cup olive oil
4 cups chicken broth (or 4 bouillon cubes, dissolved in 4 cups water)
Wheat or soy flour
Bread crumbs
3 egg yolks
1/4 pound mozzarella cheese, cut into 20 cubes
1/4 cup feta cheese
1 tablespoon parsley, minced
1/8 tablespoon freshly ground pepper
1/4 teaspoon grated nutmeg

1. Prepare rice (basic recipe).
2. In a large bowl, beat 1 egg yolk. Add rice along with cheese, parsley, pepper, nutmeg. Blend well. Cover mixture and refrigerate at least 1 hour, until chilled.
3. In a small bowl, beat 2 egg yolks with 2 teaspoons water; set aside.
4. Scoop mixture. Place mozzarella in center. Shape rice with the palms of your hands into balls (1 1/2 inches) on a baking sheet. Roll balls in flour. Roll balls in egg yolks. Coat balls with bread crumbs. Place rice balls around the mozzarella. Cover with plastic wrap. Refrigerate for 2 hours.
5. In a heavy saucepan heat 3 inches of oil to 375°F. Place chilled rice balls in hot oil. Fry, occasionally turning, for 3–5 minutes, until golden brown. Remove with a spoon. Drain on paper towels. Serve at once.

Rice Piazza San Marco

Rice (basic recipe)
A&B White Sauce (basic recipe)
1 cup raisins, soaked in water for 5 hours
1/2 cup almonds, chopped
Walnuts

1. Prepare rice; set aside.
2. Prepare A&B White Sauce. Mix rice with white sauce. Add raisins and almonds. Mix well. Garnish with walnuts.

Mediterranean Rice with Broccoli

Rice (basic recipe)
1 bunch fresh broccoli, stems cut off
1/2 cup chopped olives, black and green
1/2 pound Canadian bacon, chopped
3 cloves garlic, minced or pressed
1/4 cup dry white wine
7-oz can chicken broth (or bouillon cubes)
1 cup A&B White Sauce
2 tablespoons butter
1/2 cup olive oil
1/2 cup fresh parsley, chopped
1 tablespoon basil

1. Prepare rice. Remove from heat. Place in a warm bowl.
2. Prepare A&B White Sauce.
3. In a saucepan, lightly brown oil, garlic, and bacon for 10 minutes. Add wine and let simmer over medium heat for 5 minutes. Add chicken broth and A&B White Sauce; simmer for 5 minutes. Add olives, basil, parsley, and butter; simmer another 3 minutes. Mix with rice. Mix well.

Gilbert's Rice Salad   4 servings

1 cup natural (brown) rice
4 cups lettuce (or any other greens), chopped
1 tomato, quartered
1 medium onion, quartered
1/2 cup green olives, sliced
1/2 cup walnuts, chopped
1 tablespoon olive oil
Vinegar to taste
1 teaspoon dried basil
1 teaspoon dried oregano
Sea salt to taste
Cayenne pepper to taste
Pepper to taste

1. Prepare rice (basic recipe). Let stand until rice is cool enough to be refrigerated. Refrigerate 1 hour.
2. Add lettuce, onion, tomato, olives, oil, vinegar, walnuts, basil, oregano. Season to taste. Mix well.

COUSCOUS "A"

Couscous Tunisian   4 servings

2 cups couscous
3 medium potatoes, cut in quarters
2 pounds pumpkin pulp or squash, cut in cubes
5 carrots, cut in halves
2 celery stalks, cut 3 to 4-inches long
1 green pepper
1 red pepper
2 cloves garlic
1 large onion,
1 bunch coriander, sliced
Dried coriander
Cumin
Saffron
Sea salt
Pepper
3 vegetable, beef, or chicken bouillon cubes (diluted with 3 cups of water)
Butter
Oil

1. In a large frying pan, cook onions in oil, stirring occasionally, until tender. Add pumpkin or squash. Add garlic, coriander, vegetables, salt, pepper, dried coriander, cumin, and saffron. Let cook; stir occasionally. Add 3 cups bouillon. Let cook, until tender; set aside.
2. In a vegetable steamer, place couscous over boiling water, 30 minutes. Cook until tender. Remove from heat but keep warm.
3. In a big bowl, place couscous. Pour vegetables and sauce over couscous. Serve warm.

SOUPS "A"

Classic Potato Soup   4 servings

8 potatoes (medium to large), chopped in cubes
6–7 cups (distilled) water
2 tablespoons butter
1 teaspoon olive oil
1 large onion, chopped
1 clove garlic, minced
2 cups celery, chopped
4 cups vegetable bouillon (OPTIONAL: 4 bouillon cubes)
1/4 teaspoon dried tarragon
1/2 teaspoon dried sage
1 teaspoon dried thyme
1 dash cayenne pepper
1 dash nutmeg
1 dash sea salt

In a large saucepan, melt butter and heat oil. Add onion, garlic, celery, potatoes, bouillon, and spices. Add bouillon to cover vegetables. Bring to a boil. Simmer until vegetables are soft, for 20 minutes. Mash vegetables and potatoes. Serve warm.

Corn Soup   4 servings

2 fresh ears of corn (or one 10-ounce package frozen whole
  kernel corn, thawed)
1/4 cup onion, chopped
1 clove garlic, minced
1 tablespoon butter
1 cup chicken broth (or bouillon cube)
Bottled hot sauce to taste
1/2 cup heavy cream
1/2 cup sour cream
1/4 teaspoon sea salt
1/8 teaspoon pepper
Cilantro, chopped
Parsley, chopped

1. If using fresh corn, use a sharp knife to cut off just the kernel
   tips. Then scrape the cob with a knife.
2. In a blender container or food processor combine half of the
   corn, sour cream, and heavy cream. Cover and blend or process
   until smooth, stopping machine occasionally to scrape down
   sides. Set mixture aside.
3. In a medium saucepan, cook onion and garlic in butter until
   tender but not brown. Stir in mixture, remaining corn, broth,
   salt, pepper, and hot pepper sauce. Bring to boiling. Reduce heat
   and simmer for 20–25 minutes. Gradually stir in cream. Heat
   through, but do not boil. Season to taste. Garnish with parsley
   and cilantro.

DESSERTS "A"

Banana Cream

2 pounds bananas
2 cups heavy cream, whipped
1/2 teaspoon vanilla
1/4 cup almonds, minced
Honey to taste
Raisins to taste

> In a processor, combine bananas with whipped cream and 1/2 teaspoon vanilla. Process until mixture is firm. Garnish with raisins; sprinkle almonds over banana cream; refrigerate.

Fried Bananas

Bananas, cut in halves
Butter to taste
Almonds, chopped
2 tablespoons honey

> In a frying pan, cook butter until golden brown. Add bananas. Fry until golden brown. Remove pan from heat. Sprinkle nuts, almonds, and honey over banana. Serve immediately.

Banana Flambé

1 banana, sliced
2 tablespoons honey
2 tablespoons butter
Cognac to taste
Walnuts, chopped
Almonds, chopped

> In a frying pan, place banana. Top with nuts and almonds. Fry until golden brown. Add butter. Let cook until melted. Add cognac. Burn alcohol. Serve flambé with nuts.

Dessert "Amadeus Mozart"

1 cup cottage cheese (or ricotta cheese)
1/2 cup soaked raisins for 5 hours
1/2 cup heavy cream, whipped
2 egg yolks (*)
1/8 cup hazelnuts

In a medium bowl, combine ingredients. Mix well. Refrigerate.

(*)There is some danger of salmonella from uncooked egg yolk.

ICE CREAM "A"

Banana Ice Cream

2 cups heavy cream, whipped
1 pound bananas
2 tablespoons honey
1/2 cup walnuts, crushed

1. In a processor, combine whipped cream with fruit. Sweeten to taste.
2. In a plastic bowl, put mixture into freezer and chill at least 1 to 1-1/2 hours. Serve with whipped cream and decorate with walnuts.

Vanilla Ice Cream–Frozen Custard

2 cups heavy cream, whipped
4 egg yolks (*)
2 tablespoons honey
1 teaspoon vanilla
Walnuts

1. In a processor combine whipped cream with egg yolks, honey, and vanilla. Process until mixture is foaming.
2. In a plastic bowl, put mixture into freezer and chill for at least 1 to 1-1/2 hours. Serve with whipped cream and decorate with walnuts.

(*)There is some danger of salmonella from uncooked egg yolks.

Nut Ice Cream

2 cups heavy cream, whipped
4 egg yolks (*)
2 tablespoons honey
2 cups hazelnuts, crushed

1. In a processor combine whipped cream with egg yolks, honey, and hazelnuts. Process, until mixture is foaming.
2. In a plastic bowl, put mixture into freezer and chill at least for 1 to 1-1/2 hours. Serve with whipped cream and decorate with hazelnuts.

(*)There is some danger of salmonella from uncooked egg yolks.

Cheese Cake

1 cup whole wheat flour
4 tablespoons butter
2 egg yolks
1 cup water
1 cup heavy cream
1 tablespoon honey
4 tablespoons honey
1 1/2 pounds cottage cheese or ricotta cheese
1 package vanilla pudding powder
1 teaspoon baking powder
1/2 cup raisins

1. Preheat oven to 250°F.
2. In a large bowl, combine flour, butter, water, cream, baking powder, and honey. Knead dough well. Using a rolling pin, place dough on baking tin.
3. Combine cottage or ricotta cheese with heavy cream (or water), vanilla pudding powder, honey, egg yolks, and raisins; add baking powder and vanilla mixture. Place mixture on dough.
4. Bake cake until cheese mixture is firm.
5. Let stand 15 minutes in oven.

Blueberry Cookies

Same dough as cheese cake
1 pound blueberries

1. Preheat oven to 300°F.
2. Knead dough. Place dough on baking tin. Cut into squares. Fill each dough square with blueberries; fold over into cookies.
3. On a baking sheet, arrange cookies. Bake for 10 minutes.

Raisin Cookies

Same dough as cheese cake
1/2 pound ricotta cheese
1 cup raisins, soaked in water for 5 hours

1. Preheat oven to 300°F.
2. Combine ricotta cheese with raisins. Mix well.
3. Knead dough. Place dough on baking tin. Cut into squares and fill with mixture.
4. On a baking sheet, arrange cookies. Bake for 10 minutes.

Nut Cookies

1/4 pound rolled oats
1/4 pound butter
4 tablespoons honey
1 egg yolk
1/2 teaspoon baking powder
1/2 pound crushed hazelnuts

1. Preheat oven to 300°F.
2. Combine ingredients. Mix dough well.
3. On a baking sheet, place little portions of dough, about 1 teaspoon each. Garnish cookies with hazelnuts.
4. Bake cookies for 10 minutes, not too dark.

Banana Cake

1 cup whole wheat flour
1 teaspoon yeast
2 bananas, mashed
1/4 pound butter
3 tablespoons honey
2 egg yolks
1/4 pound walnuts, chopped

1.   Preheat oven to 300°F.
2.   Whisk butter, honey, egg yolks until foaming. Add whole wheat flour, yeast, and mashed bananas.
3.   Place mixture in a bread pan or baking pan. Sprinkle with chopped walnuts.
4.   Bake cake for 20–25 minutes. Reduce heat. Let stand 2 minutes. Remove from heat; cut in pieces. Let cool.

Honey Pancakes

1/4 cup oil
2 egg yolks
2 cups whole wheat flour
1/2 teaspoon baking soda
1 pinch salt
1 1/2–2 cups water
1/2 pound ricotta or cottage cheese
1/2 cup raisins
1 tablespoon honey

1. Beat the egg yolks and oil together.
2. Combine flour, soda, and salt. Add to eggs.
3. Add water until batter is of desired consistency. Make pancakes on a hot griddle or frying pan coated with a little oil.
4. For topping, combine cheese, honey and raisins. Serve over pancakes.

BREAD "A"

Flat Bread
(Makes 10 flat breads)

1 pound whole wheat flour
2 teaspoons yeast
1 teaspoon sea salt
5–6 tablespoons sunflower oil
1 1/2 cup water (or sour milk)
Sesame seeds (or caraway, sunflower, or poppy seeds)

1. Preheat oven to 350°F.
2. Combine ingredients, except sesame (or caraway, sunflower, or poppy) seeds. Mix well. Let stand at least 10 minutes.
3. Form bread into pancake shapes, about 6 inches in diameter; dip in seeds.
4. Arrange bread flats on a greased baking sheet.
5. Bake bread for 10–15 minutes.

A&B SANDWICHES "A"

Replace any bread with rye, whole grain, whole wheat, potato, or Canadian oat bread.

A&B Sandwich

Whole wheat roll (rye, potato bread, oat bread
Mayonnaise
Egg yolk, cooked, crumbled or chopped
Tomato, sliced
Lettuce, preferably dark or red lettuce, chopped

1. Cut roll; spread mayonnaise; sprinkle egg yolk.
2. Add sliced tomatoes and sprinkle chopped lettuce evenly.

Pita L.T. and Onion

Pita bread
Mayonnaise
Tomatoes, sliced
Lettuce, chopped
Onions, sliced

1. Cut pita bread in half; spread mayonnaise.
2. Add tomatoes, lettuce, and onions.

Tramezzini "Romana"

2 slices whole wheat bread
Mayonnaise
Egg yolk, cooked
Lettuce, chopped
Tomatoes, sliced or chopped

1. Spread the bread with mayonnaise, sprinkle egg yolk, and add lettuce, chopped.
2. Cut the bread diagonally.

A&B Fish Roll

Roll, whole wheat or rye
Marinated white herring
Onions, sliced

Cut the roll; add herring and onions.

A&B "Oktoberfest" Sandwich

Roll, whole wheat
Salami (uncooked!)
Pickles, sliced

Cut the roll, add salami, and garnish with pickle slices (bread and
butter chips).

French Roasted Bread with Garlic

Baguette, whole wheat
Olive oil
Garlic, chopped

1. Preheat oven to 300°F.
2. Cut the baguette.
3. Pour oil over baguette and sprinkle the garlic evenly.
4. Toast the baguette in the oven.

B.L.T. Sandwich
(Either with Bacon, or Cured or Smoked Ham)

Whole wheat bread
Lettuce, dark or red, quantity to taste
Tomato, sliced
Bacon

1. Spread the bread with mayonnaise.
2. Add lettuce, tomato, and bacon.

Sandwich "Matador"

Whole wheat bread
Mayonnaise
Sliced jalapeno pepper

   Spread the bread with mayonnaise; add jalapeno pepper.

Bavarian Chives Sandwich

Whole wheat bread, rye, potato bread
Butter
Chives, chopped

   Spread the bread with butter; sprinkle chives evenly.

Salmon (Smoked or Sushi) Sandwich

Salmon, sliced
2 slices whole wheat bread or roll
Lettuce, dark or red, chopped
1 tomato, sliced
Dill, dried
Whipped cream, fresh

   1.   Spread the bread with mayonnaise.
   2.   Add salmon slice(s).
   3.   Top with tomato slices and lettuce.
   4.   Top with fresh whipped cream.
   5.   Sprinkle dill evenly.

BREAKFAST "B"

1. Whole milk and apples. The best breakfast is indeed milk (or yogurt) with apples, because you will build a strong alkaline foundation for the day.

2. Scrambled (whole) eggs with bacon *(but without bread),* with orange juice

   OR

3. Scrambled egg yolks with bacon, *in this case, with bread* (without orange juice)

4. Ham and eggs (without bread), with orange juice

LUNCH and DINNER "B"

The following dishes can be served with any kind of vegetables (except potatoes and kale); salads; honey melon, and any kind of B-fruits; avocados with shrimp, vinegar, oil, and dill; shrimp cocktail with mayonnaise; mixed A&B salad; tuna salad; Waldorf Astoria salad; chicken salad with pineapple and mayonnaise; cheese of any kind; fruit salad; apple dessert with whipped cream; and ice cream with whipped cream and other desserts. However, for health reasons *you should eat strong acid-building cooked meat and cooked fish with base-builders (fruits, salads, vegetables).*

POULTRY "B"

Poultry should not be marinated with sugar, syrup, or sugar containing sauces. You may marinate with soy flour mixed with egg yolk.

Classic Roast Chicken   4 servings

1 whole chicken
1 medium onion, thickly sliced
1 small onion, diced
2 carrots, thickly sliced
2 zucchinis, sliced
2 tablespoons butter
2 tablespoons olive oil
1 tablespoon soy flour
1 cup chicken stock or water
1 tablespoon dried thyme
Sea salt to taste
Pepper to taste

1. Rinse and dry the chicken.
2. Preheat oven to 350°F. Season chicken liberally with salt and pepper inside and out. Put small quartered onions and thyme inside cavity and tie legs together. Rub butter all over chicken.
3. Put oil in a large oval gratin dish or shallow roasting pan. Scatter sliced onion, zucchini, and carrot around the dish. Place chicken on top.
4. Roast chicken in oven until it is golden brown.
5. Remove to a serving platter and cover with foil to keep warm.
6. Remove all but 2 tablespoons fat from pan. Place over medium heat, add soy flour, and cook, stirring, until thickened. Season with salt and pepper to taste. Strain into a gravy boat and serve with chicken.

Roast Chicken with Vegetables   4 servings

1 whole chicken, about 3 pounds
4 carrots, peeled and cut into 1-inch pieces
4 small onions, peeled and quartered
2 tablespoons butter, softened
1 pinch sea salt and pepper
1 cup (dry) white wine
1 teaspoon rosemary, crushed

1. Preheat oven to 375°F. Season chicken inside and out with salt and pepper. Place 1/2 teaspoon rosemary in cavity. Tie legs together and rub butter over skin. Place in a large roasting pan.
2. Roast chicken for 15 minutes. Arrange vegetables around chicken. Sprinkle remaining rosemary over chicken and vegetables. Pour wine over all and bake 1 hour and 15 minutes with pan drippings. Add water as soon as wine evaporates.

Roast Chicken Hawaii   4 servings

1 whole chicken, about 3 pounds
2 tablespoons butter
2 tablespoons olive oil
Pineapple, diced
1/2 teaspoon dried thyme
Sea salt and pepper to taste
Dry white wine

1. Preheat oven to 350°F. Season chicken inside and out with salt and pepper. Place 1/2 teaspoon thyme in cavity. Tie legs together and rub butter over skin. Place in a large roasting pan.
2. Roast chicken for 15 minutes. Arrange diced pineapple around chicken. Sprinkle remaining thyme over chicken. Pour dry white wine over all and bake 1 hour and 15 minutes. Add water (or cream) as soon as wine evaporates.

Roast Chicken with Lemon   4 servings

1 whole chicken
1 garlic clove, split in half
1 lemon, quartered
1 small onion, quartered
Sea salt and pepper to taste

1. Preheat oven to 350°F.
2. Rinse chicken inside and out; pat dry.
3. Season inside and out with salt and pepper. Rub garlic over the skin; then place inside cavity. Stuff lemon and onion inside cavity. Tie legs together. Place chicken, breast side up, in a roasting pan.
4. Bake 1 hour and 15 minutes, until juices run clear.

Chicken with Mushrooms   4 servings

1 roasting chicken
1/4 pound mushrooms, sliced
3 tablespoons parsley, chopped
3 tablespoons cilantro, chopped
1 egg yolk, beaten
2 tablespoons chopped parsley
2 teaspoons grated lemon peel
1 tablespoon fresh lemon juice
1 garlic clove, crushed through a press
Sea salt and freshly ground pepper

1. Preheat oven to 350°F. In a large frying pan, melt 4 tablespoons of the butter over medium heat. Add onion and mushrooms and cook until onion is tender and mushrooms are lightly brown, about 5 minutes. Remove from heat. Add egg, parsley, cilantro, lemon peel, and 3/4 cup water. Mix well.
2. In a small saucepan, melt remaining 3 tablespoons butter. Add garlic and lemon juice; set aside.
3. Place chicken in a large roasting pan. Tie legs together. Season skin with salt and pepper. Brush with garlic butter.
4. Roast 2 1/2 hours, basting occasionally, until chicken is tender.

Ricotta Chicken   4 servings

1 roasting chicken, about 5 pounds, backbone removed
1 cup ricotta cheese
5 tablespoons butter
1 large onion, chopped
2 cups grated zucchini
1 garlic clove, crushed through a press
1 egg, beaten
1 teaspoon sea salt
1/2 teaspoon freshly ground pepper
1 teaspoon dried basil
1/2 teaspoon dried oregano
1/2 teaspoon dried marjoram

1. Preheat oven to 350°F. Flatten chicken and place in a large roasting pan, skin side up. Starting at the breast, gently pull skin away from meat.
2. In a large frying pan, melt 3 tablespoons of the butter over medium heat. Add onion and cook until tender, about 3 minutes. Add zucchini and cook until wilted, about 3 minutes longer; remove from heat.
3. Add ricotta cheese, marjoram, egg, salt, and pepper. Mix well.
4. Spoon stuffing under the skin working over breast, thigh, and leg areas, smoothing it evenly under skin.
5. In a small saucepan, melt remaining 2 tablespoons butter. Add garlic, basil, and oregano. Brush chicken with seasoned butter. Roast 1-1/2 hours until tender and juices run clear, basting every 20 or 30 minutes.

Parmesan Chicken   4 servings

1 chicken, 3 pounds, cut up
3 tablespoons butter
2 tablespoons soy flour
1 cup sweet cream (diluted with water)
1/2 cup grated Parmesan cheese
1/2 cup shredded Swiss cheese
Sea salt and pepper

1. Preheat oven to 350°F. Season chicken with salt and pepper. In a large frying pan, melt butter over medium heat. Add chicken and cook, turning, until brown, about 10 minutes.
2. Sprinkle 1/4 cup of the Parmesan cheese over bottom of a medium baking dish. Arrange chicken in dish.
3. In same frying pan, whisk soy flour into pan drippings. Cook, stirring, for 1 minute. Gradually add cream and cook, stirring constantly, until smooth and thick. Remove from heat and stir in Swiss cheese. Pour sauce over chicken.
4. Top chicken with remaining 1/4 cup Parmesan cheese. Bake for 45 minutes, until chicken is tender.

Chicken with Spinach   4 servings

2 cups chopped cooked chicken
3 tablespoons butter
3 tablespoons soy flour
1 3/4 cups cream (with water)
1 pound spinach, chopped
1 cup grated Parmesan cheese
10 slices Swiss cheese
1/2 pound mushrooms, halved
1 teaspoon sea salt
1 teaspoon pepper
1/4 teaspoon nutmeg
2 tablespoons water
Paper towels

1. Preheat oven to 350°F. Place spinach in a large saucepan with 2 tablespoons water. Cover and steam until tender, about 3 minutes. Drain well; press between paper towels to squeeze out excess water. Transfer to a medium baking dish.
2. In a large saucepan, melt butter over medium heat. Stir in flour and cook, without browning, for 1 minute. Gradually whisk in cream and soy flour. Add salt, pepper, and nutmeg. Cook, stirring constantly, until mixture thickens and comes to a boil. Reduce heat to low, add Swiss cheese, and cook until melted.
3. Remove sauce from heat. Add chicken and mushrooms. Pour over spinach.
4. Sprinkle Parmesan cheese over chicken. Bake for 20 minutes, until bubbly and lightly brown on top.

Chicken Thighs with Vegetables   4 servings

8 pieces chicken thighs
1/2 cup grated Parmesan cheese
2 tablespoons butter
4 tablespoons butter, melted
1 cup grated carrots
1 cup broccoli, chopped
1 onion, chopped
Sea salt to taste
Pepper to taste
Oregano to taste

1. Preheat oven to 350°F. Place chicken on a baking sheet. Sprinkle the chicken with butter and Parmesan cheese. Bake until chicken is tender, for 45 minutes.
2. In a frying pan, melt butter over medium-high heat. Add carrots, broccoli, and onion and cook, tossing often, 5 minutes, until broccoli is crisp-tender.
3. Serve chicken mixed in with vegetables.

Chicken Wings and Blue Cheese Dip   4 servings

24 whole chicken wings
2–4 cups olive oil
4 tablespoons butter
2–5 tablespoons hot pepper sauce
1 tablespoon distilled white vinegar
Celery sticks
Sea salt and pepper

1. Rinse chicken and pat dry. Cut off and discard pointed tip of each wing and halve wings at the main join. Season chicken with salt and pepper to taste. In a large, heavy saucepan, heat 2 inches of oil to 375°F on a deep-frying thermometer. Cook the wings, in batches without crowding, until crisp and golden, about 10 minutes. Drain well on paper towels.
2. In a small saucepan, melt butter over medium-low heat. Stir in hot sauce and vinegar. Mound wings on a serving plate and pour hot butter sauce over them. Serve at once, with celery sticks and blue cheese dip.

Chicken with Herbs   4 servings

1 chicken, 3 pounds, cut up
2 tablespoons butter
2 tablespoons chopped onion
2 tablespoons chopped parsley
1/2 cup dry white wine
1/4 cup grated Parmesan cheese
1 teaspoon paprika
1/4 teaspoon dried marjoram
1/4 teaspoon dried tarragon
1/2 teaspoon poultry seasoning
1/2 teaspoon dried oregano

1. Preheat oven to 350°F. In a small saucepan, melt butter over medium heat. Add onion and cook until tender, about 3 minutes. Stir in parsley, oregano, poultry seasoning, tarragon, marjoram, and wine. Boil 5 minutes, until sauce is reduced by one-third.
2. Arrange chicken in a medium baking dish. Brush herb sauce over chicken. Sprinkle with Parmesan cheese and paprika. Bake 45 minutes, until tender.

Classic Baked Chicken   4 servings

1 whole chicken, 3 pounds, cut up
2 large garlic bulbs, separated into cloves
3 celery stalks, cut into 1-inch lengths
1/4 cup olive oil
1/4 cup dry white wine
2 tablespoons parsley, chopped
2 tablespoons fresh basil, chopped, or 1/4 teaspoon dried
1/4 tablespoon freshly ground pepper
1/4 teaspoon hot pepper, crushed
3 tablespoons fresh lemon juice and 1/2 teaspoon grated lemon rind
Sea salt to taste

1. Preheat oven to 375°F. Arrange chicken in a medium baking dish, skin side up. Sprinkle garlic cloves and celery over chicken.
2. Mix wine, oil, salt, pepper, basil, lemon juice, and hot pepper. Pour over chicken. Sprinkle lemon rind on top.
3. Bake, covered, for 40 minutes. Uncover and bake 15 minutes, until chicken is tender.

Chicken Veneziana   4 servings

2 chickens (about 3 pounds each), quartered
6 tablespoons butter
1/2 cup grated white Cheddar cheese
1 can (28 ounces) Italian peeled tomatoes, drained and finely chopped
1 1/4 cups soy flour
2 cups cream
2 tablespoons olive oil
3 large onions, sliced
1/4 pound boiled ham, cut into thick strips
1/2 teaspoon white pepper and 1/4 teaspoon black pepper
1 teaspoon dried basil

1. Preheat oven to 350°F. In a saucepan, melt 4 tablespoons of the
    butter over medium heat. Whisk in 1/4 cup of the soy flour and
    cook, stirring, 2 minutes without browning. Gradually whisk in
    cream. Bring to a boil and cook, stirring, until thickened; season
    with white pepper. Remove from heat and stir in Cheddar
    cheese.
2. Place remaining 1 cup soy flour and black pepper in plastic bag.
    Add chicken quarters and shake to coat. In a large frying pan,
    melt remaining 2 tablespoons butter in oil over medium heat.
    Brown chicken in pan in batches, about 4 minutes on each side;
    remove to a large roasting pan.
3. Add onions to frying pan and cook 3 minutes, until softened.
    Add ham, tomatoes, cheese, sauce and basil. Cook 5 minutes.
    Pour sauce over chicken and cover. Bake 1 hour.
4. Arrange chicken on a large heated platter. Coat lightly with
    sauce. Pass remaining sauce separately.

Chicken Liver   4 servings

1 pound chicken livers
2 tablespoons butter
2 tablespoons olive oil
2 hard-cooked egg yolks
2 medium onions, chopped
1 teaspoon minced garlic
1 teaspoon lemon juice
1/2 teaspoon freshly ground pepper
1 teaspoon sea salt

1. Trim chicken livers.
2. Broil chicken livers about 4 inches from heat, turning frequently, until brown outside and no longer pink inside, 5–10 minutes.
3. Meanwhile, in a large skillet, cook onions in butter over medium heat until golden brown, about 10 minutes.
4. Scrape onions and olive oil into a food processor.
5. Add liver, salt, and pepper and pulse until coarsely chopped. Add eggs (or egg yolks) and chop to desired consistency. Drizzle lemon juice.

Serve with French green beans and butter.

Diced Chicken   4 servings

2 cups diced cooked chicken
2 tablespoons butter
2 tablespoons soy flour
1 cup cream (diluted with water), heated
1/2 cup cream
2 tablespoons (dry) sherry
2 egg yolks, beaten
1/2 teaspoon sea salt
1/4 teaspoon white pepper
Dash of hot pepper sauce
1 pinch celery salt

1. Melt butter in a saucepan over medium heat. Stir in flour and cook about 2 minutes, stirring constantly, without browning.
2. Gradually whisk in 1 cup cream (diluted with water) and bring to a boil, stirring constantly, until mixture thickens. Reduce heat to low. Add white pepper, salt, hot pepper sauce.
3. Whisk in 1/2 cup cream. Add sherry and chicken. Season with additional salt and white pepper to taste. Cook until hot. Remove from heat. Whisk in egg yolks, blending well, and serve.

Chicken Nuggets   4 servings

2 1/2 pounds skinless, boneless chicken breasts, cut into 1-inch pieces
Olive oil
1/2 cup cream
1/4 cup soy flour
1/4 cup grated Parmesan cheese
1 teaspoon paprika
1/2 teaspoon oregano

1. In a large frying pan, heat 1 inch of oil to 350°F.
2. Meanwhile, put cream in a bowl. In a paper bag, combine flour, Parmesan cheese, paprika, and oregano. Mix well. First dip chicken pieces in cream; then place about a dozen pieces of chicken at a time in bag and shake until they are evenly coated.
3. Fry chicken in hot oil in batches, turning occasionally, for about 5 minutes, until crisp and golden brown. Drain on paper towels, serve hot.

MINCED MEAT "B"

Minced Meat St. Tropez   4 servings

1 1/2 pounds ground beef
1 1/2 pounds vegetables (carrots, celery, tomatoes, onions), sliced
1 egg
1 cup bouillon (or vegetable water or regular water)
1 tablespoon butter (or vegetable or olive oil)
1/4 teaspoon cayenne pepper
1 pinch celery salt
1 pinch nutmeg

1. In a small frying pan, combine butter and onions until lightly brown. Add vegetables and bouillon (or vegetable water or water); cook until vegetables are tender.
2. In a small bowl, combine ground beef, egg, salt, and pepper. Mix well.
3. Roll ground beef (1/2-inch) on aluminum wrap. Place vegetables in center of meat. Fold over vegetables with meat.
4. Preheat oven to 350°F. Place meat on baking sheet. Bake meat until tender, approximately 30 minutes. Remove from heat, cut in slices, and serve with salad.

French Cabbage Roll   4 servings

1 large white cabbage
2 pounds ground beef
1/2 pound mushrooms (optional)
2 whole eggs
1/2 cup sour cream
3 large onions, chopped
1 clove garlic, crushed through a press
4 tablespoons butter or olive oil
1 pinch thyme
1 pinch cumin and fennel herbs
1 pinch pepper and 1 pinch sweet Hungarian or other paprika
1 pinch sea salt

1. Place cabbage in a vegetable steamer, for 5–7 minutes (or in boiling water). Cook until leaves are tender when pierced with tip of sharp knife. Separate tender leaves. Cut leaves in quarters.
2. In a small frying pan, cook onions until golden brown.
3. In a big bowl, combine beef, onions, eggs, and spices. Mix well.
4. On a big plate, arrange leaves and form mixture into balls. Arrange beef mixture on prepared cabbage leaves. Wrap cabbage around meat. Bind each with string.
5. In a large frying pan, melt 4 tablespoons of butter over medium heat. Add onions, and cabbage rolls. Cook cabbage rolls, turning, until brown. When golden brown, add sour cream and 1/2 cup of water. Let stand on slow fire, 45 minutes. Serve warm.

Farmer's Meat Balls   4 servings
(With Green Peas and Carrots)

1 pound ground beef
1 large onion, cut in halves
1 large onion, peeled and quartered
2 tablespoons soy flour
1 egg
2 cloves garlic, chopped
1 tablespoon butter
1/4 cup capers and laurels to taste
1 pinch herb salt and 1 pinch pepper
1 cup vegetable broth

1. In a large bowl, combine ground beef with egg and spices, until blended. Mix well. Form meat-balls.
2. In medium saucepan, bring 1 cup vegetable broth to a boil. Add 1 onion (cut in halves), laurels, garlic, and meatballs. Cook on medium heat, for 10 minutes.
3. In a medium frying pan, melt 1 tablespoon butter over medium heat. For the sauce, combine soy flour, 1 cup vegetable water, sour cream, and capers. Mix until well blended. Simmer until a thick sauce is formed. Serve with green peas and carrots.

"Veggie" Stuffed Green Peppers (OPTIONAL: Tomatoes or Zucchini)

4 servings

2 pounds ground beef
2 middle-size onions, sliced
2 middle-size onions, cut in halves
8 green peppers (or 8 zucchini or 8 large tomatoes)
5 cloves garlic, crushed through the press
   (optional: 2 teaspoons garlic powder)
1/2 bunch parsley, chopped
1/2 bunch cilantro, chopped
1/2 bunch dill, chopped
1 large lemon, juice of
2 tablespoons butter (or olive oil)
1 cup sour cream
1 cup of water
1 bouillon cube (beef, chicken, or vegetable)
1 pinch celery salt
1 pinch cumin
1 pinch cayenne pepper
1 pinch saffron

1. In a food processor or blender combine parsley, cilantro, garlic, and dill. Process until a puree forms.
2. In a big bowl, combine meat, eggs, puree, and spices (except saffron and lemon). Blend well.
3. With a sharp knife, cut off green pepper tops. Carefully remove seeds and veins, leaving stems intact.
4. Stuff green pepper with mixture.
5. Preheat oven to 350°F. On a large baking sheet, melt 2 tablespoons butter (or olive oil); bake 1 onion, cut in halves, until softened. Arrange vegetables.
6. In a small frying pan, cook 1 cup of water and add 1 bouillon cube, saffron, and lemon juice. Add to vegetables. Bake until vegetables absorb most of the juice. Remove from oven. Add sour cream. Let stand 20 minutes. Serve warm.

Meatballs

2 pounds ground beef
2 onions, chopped
2 onions, sliced
2 celery stalks, minced (food processor)
3–4 cloves garlic
1/2 bunch parsley
1 large can Italian peeled tomatoes
Butter to taste
Soy sauce to taste
Sea salt to taste
Pepper to taste
Celery salt to taste
Oregano to taste
Basil to taste

1. In a food processor or blender combine chopped onions, celery stalks, garlic, parsley, salt, pepper, celery salt, oregano, and basil. Process vegetables. Add meat and spices. Process until a puree forms. Form meatballs.
2. In a frying pan, combine butter and sliced onions until lightly brown. Add salt, pepper, oregano, parsley. celery salt, basil. Mix well. Add Italian peeled tomatoes; chop while cooking. Add meatballs and cook (low), turning, about 1 hour. Add soy sauce to taste.

MEAT "B"

Beef with Cabbage à la Napoli   4 servings

3 pounds ground beef
1 large white cabbage, sliced
1 cup shredded mozzarella cheese
1 medium onion, chopped
1/2 cup olive oil
1 can (14 ounces) Italian peeled tomatoes
1 can (8 ounces) tomato sauce
1/2 cup soy flour
1 teaspoon sea salt
1 teaspoon celery salt and 1 teaspoon sea salt
2 teaspoons caraway seeds
2 apples, peeled, cored and chopped

1. In a paper or plastic bag, mix soy flour, sea salt, and caraway seeds. Add meat, a bit at a time, and shake until evenly coated.
2. In a large frying pan, heat oil over medium heat. Add meat preparation and cook, turning, until cooked. Transfer to a medium baking dish.
3. Preheat oven to 350°F. In the same pan, cook onion about 3 minutes, until tender. Add tomatoes, tomato sauce, apples, sea salt. Bring to a boil. Add cabbage and mix well. Spoon mixture over meat.
4. Cover with foil and bake 1 hour, until meat is tender. Remove foil; sprinkle mozzarella cheese over meat. Return to oven for about 5 minutes, until cheese melts.

Zurich "Geschnetzeltes"   4 servings

1 1/2 pounds beef or veal
1 pound mushrooms, sliced
1 can green peas, drained
2 cups heavy cream
Butter to taste
2 large onions, chopped
4 cloves garlic, crushed through a press
Celery salt to taste
Garlic powder to taste
Sea salt to taste
Pepper to taste

1. Cut meat in 1/2-inch slices. Season with celery salt and pepper.
2. In a small frying pan, combine butter, onions and garlic until lightly brown. Add meat and cook, turning, until brown. Reduce heat and add mushrooms, spices and heavy cream. Cook, stirring occasionally, about 1 hour. Add peas and season to taste.

Cotoletta Milanese   4 servings

1/2 pound ground beef or veal cutlets
8 oz. cream cheese
Butter
1 pinch nutmeg
1 pinch onion powder
1 pinch sea salt
1 pinch pepper
1 pinch celery salt
1 lemon, juice of

1. Season both sides of meat to taste.
2. In a frying pan, melt butter over medium heat. Add meat. Cook, turning, until golden brown, approximately 10 minutes. Top with lemon juice.
3. Cut cream cheese into 1/8-inch slices and arrange over meat. Serve with vegetables and salad.

King Arthur's Roast with Red Cabbage)   4 servings

5–6 pound roast beef, sliced
2 large onions, sliced
5 cloves garlic, crushed through a press
4 laurels
2 cups sour (or heavy) cream
3 tablespoons olive oil
4 cups water
1 bouillon cube (vegetable, chicken, or beef)
Red wine to taste

In a frying pan, cook onions, oil, and garlic until brown. Add meat and red wine. Cook for 2 minutes. Add 4 cups of water and 1 bouillon cube. Cook meat, covered, occasionally stirring, until tender. Add sour (or heavy) cream. Serve with red cabbage and salad.

Austrian Meat Hotchpotch   4 servings

2 pounds beef, diced
2 large onions, sliced
2 large zucchinis, sliced
4 large carrots, sliced
1 eggplant, diced
1 clove garlic, minced
2 tomatoes, coarsely chopped
1 cup sour cream
2 bunch leeks, chopped
1 bunch cilantro, chopped
3 tablespoons butter
1/4 teaspoon sea salt
1 pinch pepper
1 pinch celery salt
1 pinch garlic powder

In a large frying pan, melt 3 tablespoons butter over medium heat. Add onions and cook until golden brown, about 5 minutes. Add meat, turning, until brown. Add vegetables and garlic. Cook, covered, over medium heat. Season with salt and pepper to taste. Add fresh sour cream.

GRILLED DISHES
AND STEAKS
"B"

T-bone steak, sirloin steak, beef ribs, prime ribs, and any kind of grilled dishes should not be marinated with syrup or sauces containing sugar. You can marinate with natural products like lemon, vinegar, wine, cognac, garlic powder, celery salt, sea salt, or pepper or dress with soy flour, mixed with egg yolks.

T-bone steak, sirloin steak, and any other steak and grilled dishes can be served with grilled tomatoes, onions, pepper, zucchini, mushrooms, and any other vegetable (except potatoes and kale); fried eggs and sour cream with (or without) chives; herb butter; or any other dip that doesn't contain sugar (see recipes).

Hors d'oeuvres, like avocados with shrimp, are perfect. The dish can be completed with "A&B Power Salad" or any other salads, fruit salad, apple dessert, or any other fruit dessert with whipped cream or ice cream (see recipes).

FISH "B"

The following dishes can be served with mixed salads, vegetables, "B"-fruits and Neutral fruits (NO fruits from the "A" group), and all kind of cheeses. Avocados with shrimp, lemon and dill; shrimp cocktail with mayonnaise, mozzarella with tomatoes, vinegar, oil, pepper, and salt are all great hors d'oeuvres. However, for health reasons, you should eat cooked fish with (fresh) base-building foods.

Fillet of Flounder with Vegetables   4 servings

4 flounder fillets, about 5 ounces each
2 tablespoons butter
2 medium carrots, cut into 1/4-inch dice
2 ounces green beans, stemmed, stringed and cut into long, thin strips (about 2 dozen)
1/4 cup (dry) white wine or water
1/2 teaspoon salt
1/4 teaspoon pepper

1. Preheat oven to 425°F. Arrange fish flat in a single layer in a medium baking dish. Season with salt and pepper; set aside.
2. In a small saucepan, melt butter over low heat. Add carrots, cover, and cook until slightly softened, 3–5 minutes. Stir in peas; cover and cook 1 minute longer. Remove cover and pour in wine. Bring to a boil.
3. Pour vegetable mixture over fish and cover dish loosely with aluminum foil. Bake 10 minutes, until fish is firm and opaque throughout.

Halibut Parmesan   4 servings

2 pounds fresh halibut steaks, cut 1 inch thick
3 tablespoons olive oil
1 medium onion, finely chopped
1 1/2 pounds fresh plum tomatoes, seeded and coarsely chopped,
    OR
1 (14-ounce) can Italian peeled tomatoes, drained and chopped
2 teaspoons chopped fresh oregano or 1 teaspoon dried
1/4 teaspoon salt
1/8 teaspoon pepper
1 tablespoon tomato paste (optional)
1/2 cup grated Parmesan cheese

1. Heat 2 tablespoons vegetable/olive oil in a medium saucepan.
    Add onion and cook until softened but not brown, 3–5 minutes.
    Stir in tomatoes and season with oregano, salt, and pepper. Stir
    in tomato paste for a deeper flavor, if desired. Reduce heat to
    medium-low and simmer, stirring frequently, until sauce is
    slightly thickened, about 10 minutes. Let cool slightly; then
    transfer to a food processor. Puree until smooth.
2. Preheat oven to 450°F. Pour tomato sauce into baking dish.
    Arrange fish on top. Grate Parmesan cheese and drizzle evenly
    over fish.
3. Bake 15 minutes until fish is opaque throughout. Serve at once.

Baked Whitefish with Tomato   4 servings

1 pound whitefish fillets
1 cup celery stalks, chopped
2 small carrots, chopped
1 (28-ounce) can Italian peeled tomatoes, drained and coarsely chopped
1 medium onion, chopped
2 tablespoons olive oil
2 pounds fresh spinach
1/2 plus 1/8 teaspoon salt and 1/4 teaspoon pepper

1. In a large saucepan, combine carrots, onion, and celery. Stir in
    olive oil and cook over medium heat until vegetables are
    softened, 5–7 minutes. Add tomatoes, 1/2 teaspoon salt, and

pepper. Cook over medium heat, stirring occasionally, until thick and pulpy, about 10 minutes. Transfer to a food processor and puree tomato sauce until smooth.

2. If using fresh spinach, plunge leaves in a large pot of rapidly boiling salted water. Return to a boil and immediately drain. Rinse under cold running water. If using frozen spinach, cook according to package directions. Use your hands to squeeze out excess moisture from spinach; coarsely chop.

3. Preheat oven to 425°F. Spread chopped spinach over bottom of a buttered medium baking dish. Cut whitefish crosswise into 1/2-inch-thick slices. Layer over spinach and season the remaining 1/8 teaspoon salt. Spread tomato sauce over fish. Cover dish loosely with aluminum foil. Bake 10 minutes, or until sauce is bubbly and fish is firm and white. Serve at once.

Baked Sole with Orange   4 servings

1 1/2 pounds sole fillets
1/2 teaspoon salt
1/4 teaspoon pepper
1/4 cup fresh orange juice
1 teaspoon soy flour
1/4 cup fresh orange juice
1/4 cup fresh lemon juice
1 whole orange

1. Arrange fish in a baking dish large enough to hold fillets flat in a single layer. Season with salt and pepper. Add orange juice and lemon juice. Cover and refrigerate 1 hour.

2. Use a serrated knife to cut away peel from orange. Cut between membranes to remove whole sections. Place in a small bowl and set aside.

3. Preheat oven to 425°F. Remove fish from refrigerator and cover dish tightly with aluminum foil. Bake 8–10 minutes, until firm and opaque throughout.

4. Transfer fillets to serving plates. Pour cooking liquid into a small saucepan. Dissolve soy flour in 2 tablespoons cold water. Stir into liquid in saucepan and bring to a boil over medium-high heat, stirring until thickened, for 1 minute. Spread sauce over fillets; garnish with orange slices.

Sole Meuniere   4 servings

4 sole fillets, 4 to 6 ounces each
1/2 cup soy flour
1/2 cup cream
4 tablespoons butter
2 tablespoons olive oil
2 tablespoons chopped parsley
1/2 teaspoon salt
1/4 teaspoon pepper
1 tablespoon fresh lemon

1. In a shallow bowl, combine soy flour, salt, and pepper. Dip sole in cream (with water), then dredge the soy flour mixture to coat.
2. In a large skillet, melt 2 tablespoons of butter in oil over medium-high heat. Shake excess soy flour off dredged fish and arrange fish in pan. Cook, turning once, until brown and crisp, about 2 minutes each side. Remove to serving plates. Drain off fat from pan.
3. Return skillet to heat and add remaining 2 tablespoons of butter, parsley, and lemon juice. Stir until butter is melted and well blended. Spoon a small amount of sauce over each fillet and serve.

Wolfish (Loup De Mere) with Mushrooms 4 servings

1 1/2 pounds wolfish fillets, cut into 4 equal pieces
1 clove garlic, minced
2 tablespoons butter
2 bunches scallions, chopped
1/4 pound mushrooms, thinly sliced
1 (28-ounce) can Italian peeled tomatoes, drained and chopped
10 large cabbage leaves, chopped
1/2 teaspoon salt
1/4 teaspoon pepper

1. Cut tough rib ends from cabbage leaves. Bring a large pot of salted water to boil over high heat. Add cabbage leaves and boil until limp, 3 to 5 minutes. Drain and rinse under cold running water; drain again. Lay flat on paper towels and pat dry.

2. In a large saucepan, melt butter over medium-high heat. Add scallions and garlic. Cook, stirring, until slightly softened, about 1 minute. Add mushrooms and tomatoes. Increase heat to high and boil, stirring often, until sauce is slightly thickened, about 3 minutes. Season with salt and pepper and set aside
3. Preheat oven to 425°F. Place 3 cabbage leaves together on a work surface, stem ends overlapping in center. Place a piece of fish in center. Season lightly with additional salt and pepper. Bring up ends and sides envelope fashion to completely cover the fish. Continue with remaining leaves and fish. Carefully transfer each to a buttered medium baking dish, placing each bundle snugly next to the other, seam side down.
4. Spread tomato-mushroom mixture over fish. Cover dish loosely with aluminum foil. Bake 10–12 minutes, or until fish is firm and sauce is bubbly.

Swordfish Steaks   4 servings

4 swordfish steaks, 4 to 6 ounces each
2 tablespoons grated Parmesan cheese
2 cloves garlic, peeled
1/3 cup olive oil
1/4 cup pine nuts
1 cup fresh basil leaves
1/4 teaspoon salt
1/8 teaspoon pepper
Lemon slices

1. Preheat oven to 425°F. Arrange fish steaks in a large, lightly oiled baking dish. In a food processor, combine basil, garlic, pine nuts, Parmesan cheese, salt, and pepper. Puree until smooth. With machine on, slowly pour in olive oil. Process until mixture is well blended.
2. Spread mixture evenly over swordfish steaks. Cover dish loosely with aluminum foil. Bake until steaks are white throughout but still moist, 10–12 minutes. Garnish with thin slices of lemon.

Swordfish (or Tuna)   4 servings

4 (1-inch-thick) swordfish (or tuna) steaks, about 6 ounces each
2 medium ripe tomatoes, peeled, seeded, and chopped
2 tablespoons vegetable or olive oil
1 small clove garlic, crushed through a press
1/2 teaspoon salt
1/4 teaspoon pepper
1 tablespoon dried thyme
1/4 cup dry white wine

1. In a large saucepan, cook swordfish (or tuna) in vegetable or olive oil over medium-high heat, turning once, 7–9 minutes. Remove to a serving platter and cover with aluminum foil to keep warm.
2. Pour off fat in pan. Add white wine, increase heat to high, and boil, stirring constantly, until reduced by half, about 1 minute. Stir in tomatoes, thyme, and garlic. Reduce heat to medium and cook, stirring often, until thick and pulpy, 3–5 minutes. Season with salt and pepper. Spoon tomato sauce over swordfish or tuna and serve.

Smoked Salmon and Parmesan   2 servings

3 ounces thinly sliced smoked salmon
1/4 teaspoon hot pepper sauce
Dash of lemon juice
8 ounces natural cream cheese, softened
1 cup fresh dill or parsley
3/4 cup grated Parmesan cheese (about 3 ounces)

1. Preheat oven to 400°F. In a small bowl or food processor, combine cream cheese, Parmesan cheese, lemon juice, and hot sauce. Blend well.
2. Cut smoked salmon into 30 pieces. Spoon about 2 teaspoons of cheese mixture over salmon and top each with dill (or parsley). Bake until cheese is just softened, about 5 minutes. Serve warm.

Shrimp   4 servings

1 1/2 pounds large shrimp
1 1/2 cups soy flour
2 tablespoons butter, melted and cooled
2 eggs, separated
1 cup olive oil
8 broccoli florets
1 small onion, sliced
1 teaspoon salt
1/2 teaspoon pepper

1. Slit shrimp down back and remove intestinal vein and shell; leave tails intact. Spread shrimp open to butterfly. Keep refrigerated until ready to cook.
2. In a large mixing bowl, combine soy flour, butter, salt, pepper, and egg yolks. Mix to form a thin batter. Cover and refrigerate for 4–6 hours.
3. When ready to cook, preheat oven to 200°F. Pour enough olive oil into a deep-fat fryer or larger saucepan. Heat to 375°F. Beat egg whites until stiff and fold into batter. In batches without crowding, dip shrimp into batter, one at a time, and drop into hot olive oil. Fry until lightly brown, 3–5 minutes. Drain on paper towels and keep warm in oven while frying vegetables.
4. Dip onion slices and broccoli florets into batter, one at a time, and fry for 1 to 1-1/2 minutes, or until coating is crisp and light beige in color. Drain on paper towels, transfer to oven to keep warm.
5. Serve shrimp with vegetables.

Chicken Soup   4 servings

5 pounds stewing chicken, cut up
6 cups (filtered) water
3 stalks celery, cut up
1 small onion, cut up
1/4 teaspoon salt
1/8 teaspoon pepper
1 bay leaf
16 ounces Italian peeled tomatoes (can), cut up
3 medium carrots, cut into julienne strips
1/2 cup onions, chopped
4 teaspoons instant chicken bouillon granules (sold in a jar)
1 cup zucchini, halved lengthwise and sliced

1. In a saucepan, combine chicken pieces, water, onion, celery, salt, pepper, and bay leaf. Bring to a boil. Reduce heat and simmer, covered, for 2 hours until chicken is tender. Remove chicken from broth. Let stand until chicken is cool enough to handle; then cut off meat and cube chicken; set aside.
2. Meanwhile, strain broth, discarding vegetables and bay leaf. Return broth to oven. Stir in tomatoes, onion, carrots, and bouillon. Simmer, covered, for 20 minutes until carrots are almost tender.
3. Add chicken to broth mixture along with zucchini. Simmer, covered, about 5 minutes until vegetables are tender.

VEGETABLES "B"

Eggplant with Tomatoes   4 servings

2 large eggplants (or 4 small)
6 cloves garlic, crushed through a press
2 medium tomatoes, pureed
4 small onions, peeled
1 cup olive oil
1 bunch parsley, chopped
1 bunch cilantro, chopped
Sea salt
Pepper
Celery salt

1. With a sharp knife, remove stem end of eggplants. Cut eggplants in 1/2-inch slices.
2. Chop cilantro and parsley. Puree tomatoes. Add garlic. Mix well.
3. In a large saucepan, heat cooking oil. Place eggplants in oil. Fry until brown.
4. Preheat oven to 300°F. On a baking sheet, place eggplants. Sprinkle tomato-cilantro-parsley mixture over eggplants. Bake for 20 minutes, until crispy. Season to taste.

SALADS "B"

Waldorf Astoria Salad

2 cups diced apples (2 medium apples)
2 sweet oranges, diced (without seeds)
1/2 pound cooked chicken, diced
3/4 cup celery, coarsely chopped
1 cup mayonnaise
1 cup sour cream
4 tablespoons heavy cream, whipped
1/2 cup coarsely chopped walnuts
1 dash cognac
2 tablespoons lemon juice (or vinegar)
1 dash salt

In medium bowl, combine all ingredients (except whipped cream, sour cream, and walnuts). Mix well. Chill thoroughly. Add whipped cream, sour cream, and walnuts before serving. Serve on lettuce. Refrigerate leftovers.

Hawaiian Chicken Salad

1/2 pound cooked chicken (or leftovers), diced
2 cups pineapple, diced
1 cup mayonnaise
Dash vinegar
Dash pepper
Pinch garlic salt
Pinch nutmeg

In medium bowl, combine all ingredients; mix well. Chill thoroughly. Serve on lettuce; top with diced pineapple.

Peking Chicken Salad

1 pound cooked (or fried) chicken (or any kind of poultry), diced
2 oranges, diced (without seeds)
1 peel of orange, grated
2 cups mayonnaise
1 cup almonds, cut in halves
Dash cognac
Pinch nutmeg

> In a large bowl, combine all ingredients; mix well. Chill thoroughly.
> Serve on lettuce; garnish with orange slices.

Carrot Salad d'Alsace

1 pound large carrots
1/4 pound cooked ham, quartered
2 oranges, juice
1 peel of orange, grated
2 cups mayonnaise
Dash garlic salt
Dash pepper
Dash nutmeg

> Cut carrots into 1/8-inch slices. Combine ham, with juice of grated
> oranges and grated peel of oranges; add mayonnaise. Mix well. Add
> to carrots. Chill thoroughly. Serve on lettuce.

Swiss Cheese Salad

1/2 pound Swiss cheese, thinly sliced
2 medium onions, thinly sliced into rings
Olive oil to taste
Vinegar to taste
Salt to taste
Pepper to taste

> In medium bowl, combine all ingredients. Add salt and pepper to
> taste. Mix well.

Sylvia's Tuna Salad

1 (6 1/2 ounce) can tuna (in oil or water)
1/4 cup capers, cut in halves
3 tablespoons onion, chopped
2 tablespoons mustard
1/2 cup pickled cucumbers, diced
1/3 cup parsley, chopped
Olive oil, quantity to taste
1 teaspoon fresh lemon juice (or vinegar)
1/4 teaspoon pepper
Salt to taste
Garlic salt to taste

In a medium bowl, mash tuna with oil and mustard. Add onions, lemon juice, pickled cucumber dices, capers, salt and pepper. Mix well. Serve on lettuce. Garnish with remaining capers, or pickled cucumber slices.

Bavarian Sausage Salad

1/2 pound Bologna sausage, sliced
2 medium onions, thinly sliced into rings
Olive oil to taste
Vinegar to taste
Salt to taste
Pepper to taste

Cut across sausage in 1/4-inch slices. Mix with onion slices. Add oil, vinegar, salt and pepper. Mix well.

Chef Salad

Lettuce (quantity to taste)
Tomatoes, sliced or diced into cubes
Cucumber, thinly sliced
Broccoli, sliced
Cauliflower, sliced
Carrots, thinly sliced
Onions, sliced or diced into cubes
1–2 boiled eggs, sliced
Swiss cheese, thinly sliced
Smoked ham, sliced
Cooked turkey or chicken, rectangularly sliced
Oil to taste
Vinegar to taste
Salt to taste
Pepper to taste
Mayonnaise (OPTIONAL: dip or dressing)

> Cut up vegetables. In a large bowl, combine all vegetables, smoked ham, and turkey or chicken. Add oil, vinegar, salt, and pepper. Add mayonnaise (or dip or dressing). Mix well.

HORS d'OEUVRE "B"

Avocados with Shrimp   1–2 servings

1 large avocado (1/2 for every person)
1 can shrimp, drained
4 tablespoons lemon juice
1 bunch dill, chopped
4 tablespoons olive oil
Salt to taste
Pepper to taste

1. Using a sharp knife, cut avocado in half. Remove pit.
2. In a medium bowl, combine lemon juice, oil, salt, and pepper to taste. Mix well.
3. Arrange shrimp on avocado. Top with dill. Pour mixture over avocado and dill. Serve immediately or cover with plastic wrap to prevent avocado from darkening. Refrigerate.

DESSERTS "B"

Creamy Fruit Dessert

1 pound strawberries, chopped
1 pound raspberries, chopped
1/2 pound peaches, chopped
2 cups heavy cream, whipped
Sweetener

Mix ingredients well and refrigerate.

Apple Dessert

5 medium apples, cored, peeled, and 1/2-inch sliced
Olive oil
Dash cinnamon powder

In a frying pan, heat oil and fry 1/2-inch apple slices until golden brown. Sprinkle cinnamon powder to taste.

Baked Apple

5 apples, peeled
1/2 cup walnuts, coarse-grained, chopped
Sweetener

1. Remove cores from apples. Fill apples with walnuts.
2. Preheat oven to 350°F. Top every apple with a piece of butter. Bake until lightly browned.

Swiss Fruit Salad

1 grapefruit, diced
2 sweet oranges, diced
2 apples, cored, peeled, and sliced in cubes
1 cup pineapple, diced
1 peel of orange, grated
2 cups whipped cream, chilled
1 dash cognac
1 dash cinnamon
Sweetener

In a large bowl, combine all ingredients. Refrigerate for 30 minutes.
Serve cool.

ICE CREAM "B"

Strawberry (Raspberry, Kiwi) Ice Cream
(Or Any Other "B"-fruit)

2 cups heavy cream, whipped
1 pound fruit

1. In a processor, combine whipped cream with fruit.
2. In a plastic bowl, put mixture into freezer and chill at least for 1–1 1/2 hours. Serve with whipped cream. Garnish with fresh fruits.

"NEUTRAL"

BREAKFAST "NEUTRAL"

The best breakfast is indeed milk (or yogurt) with apples, because you will build a strong alkaline foundation for the day. However, if you would like to eat a breakfast on a "Neutral" basis, then you will find in the following some ideas:

- Blueberries with yogurt, blueberries with cream or whipped cream

- Goat's milk cheese or ewe's milk cheese, Camembert, or any other cream cheese with vegetables, salads, and/or sprouts

- Cottage cheese or ricotta cheese with apples or any other "B" or Neutral fruit

- Cottage cheese or ricotta cheese, mixed with cream and herbs

- Smoked ham, smoked sausages, salami, beef-salami, bacon, rolled ham, or any cured, dried, or smoked meat with vegetables and/or salads

- Smoked herring, smoked mackerel, smoked salmon, or any smoked fish with vegetables and/or salads and/or dips

LUNCH
and
DINNER
"NEUTRAL"

BEANS "NEUTRAL"

Beans are believed to be difficult to digest, yet fava beans are the Egyptian national dish. The Egyptians don't have any problem digesting beans. They soak the beans for several hours in water to prepare them (unknowingly) for a chemical process that makes digestion easier. The Egyptians eat fava beans with wheat bread, olive oil, and several raw onions, radishes, and/or special salads (Ramses Salad), which are base-builders.

Ramses Beans with Ramses Salad

Old Egyptian recipe; beans should be eaten with Ramses Salad (or raw onions) to ensure proper digestion.

2 pounds small fava beans
1 pound skinless fava beans
1 pound garbanzo beans (chickpeas)
1/2 pound yellow lentils
1 large garlic bulb, crushed through a press
2 tablespoon cumin
2 tablespoon dried coriander
Salt to taste
Pepper to taste

1. Wash beans and lentils separately. In a big bowl, combine fava beans, skinless fava beans, and garbanzo beans. Cover beans with plenty of (distilled) cold water. Soak beans for 3–4 hours, or longer is best. Remove from water.
2. In a large saucepan, bring water to a boil. Add fava beans and garbanzo beans. Cover with water, 4 inches above. Reduce heat.
3. Check the water level every hour; exchange water and add water if necessary.
4. Simmer over medium-low heat for 4–5 hours, until soft. As soon as beans are soft, add lentils. Let cook, for 1 hour, until soft. Add garlic, cumin, coriander, salt, and pepper. Let stand, for 30 minutes. Serve warm; top the Ramses Beans with Ramses Salad. (OPTIONAL: mash beans with mixer. Top beans with Ramses Salad.)

Ramses Salad

(OPTIONAL: Onions, dressed with vinegar, pepper, salt, and cumin. Crush onions with your hand to enhance flavor.)

5–6 fresh hot peppers, such as jalapenos
2–3 large tomatoes
2 large onions
1 head lettuce
1 bunch cilantro
6 large cloves garlic
1 tablespoon coriander
1 tablespoon cumin
Salt to taste
Pepper to taste
1/2 cup vinegar
1/2 cup olive oil

Combine all ingredients in a food processor. Process until well blended to form a pulp. Top Ramses Beans with 3 tablespoons Ramses Salad.

TIP: In a jar, put remaining Ramses Salad. Cover with olive oil, 2 inches above pulp. Refrigerate for later use. (Also tastes great with whole wheat bread or pita.)

SOUPS "NEUTRAL"

Oriental Lentil Soup   4 servings

1 1/2 cups lentils, dried
2 cups vegetable or chicken bouillon (or cubes)
8 cups (distilled) water
1 large onion, minced
1 clove garlic, crushed through a press
2 stalks celery, chopped
2 large carrots, chopped
2 tablespoons fresh parsley, chopped
1/2 teaspoon dried thyme
1/2 teaspoon sea salt
3 tablespoons olive oil
1 teaspoon dried oregano
1 teaspoon sweet Hungarian paprika

1. In a saucepan, heat oil over medium-high setting. Add onions, tossing for 5 minutes, until crisp-tender.
2. Add garlic, carrots and celery. Add seasoning and herbs; mix well, tossing for 3–4 minutes.
3. Add vegetable or chicken bouillon; cook for 3 minutes.
4. Add lentils and 8 cups water. Simmer over low heat for about 60 minutes; add parsley.

Creamy Cauliflower Soup   4 servings

6 cups (distilled) water
2 medium cauliflowers, cored and coarsely chopped
1 onion, chopped
1 clove garlic, crushed through a press
2 tablespoons butter
1 tablespoon olive oil
2 stalks celery, chopped
8 scallions, chopped
2 tablespoons vegetable bouillon (or bouillon cubes)
1/8 teaspoon fresh ground black pepper
1/8 teaspoon nutmeg
1 teaspoon dried basil
1/2 teaspoon dried thyme
1 teaspoon dried marjoram
1/2 teaspoon celery or sea salt

In a large saucepan, melt butter and heat oil. Add scallions, onions, garlic, cauliflower and celery. Season with salt and pepper to taste. Cook over medium heat for several minutes, stirring frequently. Add water and bouillon; bring to a boil. Add basil, thyme and marjoram. Simmer, covered, over medium heat until cauliflower is tender, for 10–15 minutes. Remove cover and cool slightly. In blender, process until soup is smooth and creamy. Repeat; add nutmeg to taste.

VEGETABLES "NEUTRAL"

Broccoli Milanese   4 servings

4 stalks broccoli, washed and stems cut off
2 tablespoons butter
2 teaspoons fresh lemon juice or vinegar
Seasoning to taste

1. Cut each broccoli stem into individual florets. Place in vegetable
    steamer over boiling water until tender, covered, for 7 minutes.
2. In small saucepan, melt butter; combine with lemon juice. Pour
    sauce over hot broccoli. Season to taste.

Carrots Vienna   4 servings

12 medium carrots, peeled
3 tablespoons butter
1/4 teaspoon sea salt
2 teaspoons fresh (or dried) basil
Soy sauce

1. Cut carrots into 1/8-inch slices. Place carrots in a vegetable
    steamer over boiling water until tender, for 10 minutes. Remove
    from heat and set aside.
2. In large saucepan, melt butter. Add carrots, basil and sea salt.
    Stir well. Season to taste.

Mushrooms Lyon 4 servings

1/2 pound mushrooms
1 tablespoon butter
1 tablespoon fresh lemon juice
Dash sea salt
Dash garlic salt
Soy sauce

1. Wash mushrooms; cut ends from stems. Cut mushrooms into slices.
2. In a saucepan, melt butter. Add mushrooms, tossing lightly in butter, until soft. Add lemon juice. Season to taste.

Vegetables Parisian 4 servings

6 carrots, cut into cubes
2 medium zucchini, sliced
2 medium yellow squash
2 tablespoons butter
2 teaspoons fresh lemon juice or vinegar
Soy sauce to taste
Seasoning to taste

In a vegetable steamer, place carrots over boiling water for 10 minutes. Add zucchini and steam until tender, for 7 minutes. Arrange vegetables on a plate. Cut squash in cubes. Combine butter and lemon juice (or vinegar) and pour over vegetables. Season to taste.

Artichokes Venetian   4 servings

4 artichokes
Several celery stalks
1 bay leaf
1 clove garlic, crushed through a press

1. Wash artichokes. Trim end of stem. Snip thorny tip off each leaf. Combine garlic, celery stalks, and bay leaf.
2. In a vegetable steamer, place artichokes over boiling water, for 30–40 minutes, according to size. As soon as leaves can be removed, discard bay leaf, celery, and garlic. Serve with melted butter.

Cauliflower Soufflé Côte d'Azur   4 servings

1 large cauliflower, cored and broken into small florets
3 tablespoons olive oil
2 egg yolks
1/4 cup parsley, chopped
1 pinch sweet Hungarian paprika or other paprika
1 pinch nutmeg

1. Preheat oven to 350°F.
2. In a saucepan, cook cauliflower in boiling salted water until just tender, for 10 minutes. Remove from heat.
3. In a small soufflé dish, heat 1 tablespoon oil.
4. Whisk two egg yolks, with 2 teaspoons oil, nutmeg, pepper, and parsley.
5. Transfer cauliflower to soufflé dish
6. Spread mixture over cauliflower. Place in a broiler until soufflé is golden brown, 5–7 minutes.

Eggplants Normandy   4 servings

2 large eggplants (or 4 small)
6 cloves garlic, crushed through a press
4 small onions, peeled
2 medium tomatoes, pureed
2 cups olive oil
1 bunch parsley, chopped
1 bunch cilantro, chopped
Sea salt
Pepper
Celery salt

1. Preheat oven to 300°F.
2. With a sharp knife, remove stem end of eggplants. Cut eggplants in 1/2-inch slices.
3. Chop cilantro and parsley. Add garlic. Mix well.
4. In a large saucepan, heat cooking oil. Place eggplant in olive oil. Fry until brown.
5. On a baking sheet, place eggplant slices. Sprinkle tomato-cilantro-parsley mixture over eggplants. Bake for 20 minutes, until crispy. Season to taste.

Cabbage Budapest   4 servings

1 white cabbage, sliced
1 pound onions, diced
2 cups vegetable water (or bouillon cube)
Butter to taste
2 cups heavy cream
1 cup sour cream
2 tablespoons butter
Sea salt to taste
2 teaspoons Hungarian paprika
Soy sauce to taste

1. In a large saucepan, cook onions in butter until golden brown. Add vegetable water and sea salt to taste.
2. Place cabbage in saucepan and cook for 15–20 minutes. Remove from heat and drain.
3. Combine heavy cream and sour cream with paprika and season to taste. Sprinkle mixture over cabbage. Let stand 10 minutes.

HORS d'OEUVRES "NEUTRAL"

Mozzarella with Tomatoes   4 servings

2 large tomatoes, sliced
1 ball mozzarella, sliced
Fresh basil
Vinegar to taste
Olive oil to taste
Salt to taste
Pepper to taste

1. Cut tomatoes and mozzarella in thin slices. Arrange on a platter or serving plate.
2. In a small bowl, combine vinegar and oil. Pour mixture over mozzarella and tomatoes. Add salt and pepper to taste. Garnish with fresh basil.

Avocados with Lemon and Olive Oil   1–2 servings

1 large avocado (1/2 for every person)
4 tablespoons lemon juice
1 bunch dill, chopped
4 tablespoons olive oil
Salt to taste
Pepper to taste

1. Using a sharp knife, cut avocado in halves. Remove pit.
2. In a medium bowl, combine lemon juice, oil, salt, and pepper to taste. Mix well.
3. Top with dill. Pour mixture over avocado and dill. Serve immediately, or cover with plastic wrap to prevent avocado from darkening. Refrigerate.

OPTIONAL: Dill Dip or Creamy Avocado Dressing (see recipe "Salad Dressings & Other Dips")

SALADS "NEUTRAL"

There is no limit in quantity of vegetables, salads, sprouts, and herbs. You can add any further vegetable. Variety is important! The best vegetables to use for the purpose of detoxification are the root vegetables—carrots, turnips, and beets—and all sorts of top vegetables, such as spinach, beet tops, chard, celery, onion tops, watercress, broccoli, cauliflower, sprouts, or any green vegetable that contains juice.

A&B Power Salad

Lettuce (romaine, iceberg, limestone, red leaf, watercress, or any other
    lettuce, broken into bite-size pieces)
Tomatoes, sliced or diced into cubes
Cucumber, sliced or diced into cubes
Carrots, chopped or sliced
Cauliflower, chopped
Broccoli, chopped
White and/or red cabbage, chopped
Sprouts/soy sprouts
Spinach, chopped
Onions, sliced or diced into cubes
Scallions, sliced
Parsley, chopped
Chives, chopped
Oil to taste (olive, flaxseed, sesame, etc.)
Apple vinegar (opt: Balsamic) or fresh lemon juice to taste
Salt (sea salt, herb salt, Bio-salt) to taste
Pepper to taste

1. Cut up vegetables. In a large bowl, combine all vegetables.
2. In a small bowl, combine oil, vinegar, salt, pepper, and chives.

OPTIONAL: salad dressing, chunky blue cheese dressing, mayonnaise or dip/dressing, see section "Mayonnaise, Salad Dressing and Other Dips." Pour over salad.

Classic Green Salad

1 head lettuce—butter, red leaf, iceberg, or romaine
    (washed, dried, and sliced into bite-sized pieces)
1 small cucumber, peeled and sliced
2 tomatoes, sliced
3 carrots, sliced
1 large onion, sliced
2 garlic cloves, crushed through a press
3 tablespoons olive oil
1 tablespoon fresh lemon juice or vinegar
1/4–1/2 teaspoon sea salt
1/2 teaspoon celery salt

Place all ingredients in a bowl. Pour dressing over salad and toss well.

Ramses Salad

5–6 fresh hot peppers, such as jalapenos
2 large tomatoes
2 large onions
1 head lettuce
6 cloves garlic
1/2 cup vinegar
1/2 cup olive oil
1 tablespoon coriander
1 bunch cilantro
1 tablespoon cumin
Salt to taste
Pepper to taste

In a food processor, combine peppers, tomatoes, onions, lettuce, garlic, salt, pepper, vinegar, oil, and herbs. Process until well blended. Ideal with fava beans (see recipe "Ramses Beans"), whole wheat bread, or steamed potatoes.

Asparagus Salad

1 head lettuce
1/2 head red leaf lettuce
1/2 pound fresh (or canned) asparagus
3 tablespoons olive oil
1 tablespoon vinegar
Lemon juice to taste
1/2 teaspoon mustard
1 clove garlic, crushed through a press
Sea salt to taste
Fresh ground black pepper

1. Wash lettuce; dry and break into pieces. Break and discard heavy ends from asparagus.
2. In a medium saucepan, cook asparagus and salt in boiling salted water until tender, 3–5 minutes. Remove from water. Drain well. Cut into 1 1/2-inch pieces. Combine with lettuce.
3. For dressing, combine oil, mustard, sea salt, and lemon juice (and/or vinegar). Add pepper to taste. Mix well. Pour over salad.

Celery Salad

1 medium bunch of celery
1/2 cup mayonnaise
2 tablespoons fresh lemon juice or vinegar
2 teaspoons mustard
Seasoning to taste

1. Cut celery into very thin slices. Cut peel from slices; then julienne each slice. Add lemon juice.
2. Place celery in boiling water for 3–5 minutes until tender. Drain well. Combine mayonnaise and mustard. Toss celery in mixture. Season to taste. Serve at room temperature.

Carrot Salad

1 pound large carrots
Olive oil to taste
Lemon (or vinegar) to taste
Dash garlic salt
Dash pepper
Dash artificial sweetener

In a processor, slice carrots into 1/8-inch slices. Add remaining ingredients. Mix well. Serve on lettuce.

Cucumber with Dill

4 cucumbers, peeled and sliced
1 cup sour cream
2 tablespoons fresh lemon juice or apple vinegar
2 tablespoons fresh dill, chopped, or 1 tablespoon dried dill
1/4 teaspoon sea salt
1 teaspoon scallions, minced

Combine ingredients. Mix well.

DESSERTS "NEUTRAL"

Creamy Walnut Dessert

1 cup cottage cheese (or Ricotta cheese)
1/2 cup heavy cream, whipped
2 egg yolks (*)
1/8 cup walnuts

In a medium bowl, combine ingredients. Mix well. Refrigerate.

Creamy Blueberry Dessert

2 pounds blueberries
2 cups heavy cream, whipped
Sweetener

Mix ingredients well. Refrigerate.

(*) There is some danger of salmonella from uncooked egg yolks.

ICE CREAM "NEUTRAL"

Vanilla Ice Cream

2 cups heavy cream, whipped
4 egg yolks (*)
1 teaspoon vanilla
1 cup chopped walnuts
Artificial sweetener

1. In a processor, combine whipped cream with egg yolks, vanilla, and artificial sweetener. Process until mixture is foaming.
2. Put mixture into a plastic bowl. Put in freezer. Chill at least 1 to 1 1/2 hours. Serve with whipped cream. Garnish with walnuts.

Hazelnut Ice Cream

2 cups heavy cream, whipped
4 egg yolks (*)
2 cups hazelnuts, crushed
2 packets artificial sweetener

1. In a processor, combine whipped cream with egg yolks, hazelnuts, and artificial sweetener. Process until mixture is foaming.
2. Put mixture into plastic bowl. Put in freezer. Chill at least 1 to 1-1/2 hours. Serve with whipped cream. Garnish with hazelnuts.

(*) There is some danger of salmonella from uncooked egg yolks.

MAYONNAISE, SALAD DRESSINGS, AND OTHER DIPS "NEUTRAL"

A&B Dressing

1 cup mayonnaise
2 tablespoons horseradish

In a bowl, combine mayonnaise and horseradish. Stir until well blended.

Classic Mayonnaise

2 egg yolks (*)
2 tablespoons olive oil
1 lemon juice or vinegar
Salt to taste

In a bowl, combine ingredients (which must be refrigerated first). Add drop by drop 2 tablespoons olive oil and lemon juice. Whisk until well blended. Refrigerate until firm.

(*) *The quantity alters for 4 egg yolks, by 8 tablespoons olive oil, lemon juice, salt, and 5 tablespoons water. There is some danger of salmonella from uncooked egg yolks.*

400

French Garlic Mayonnaise

5 egg yolks (*)
5 tablespoon olive oil
5 tablespoon (filtered) water
1 lemon juice or vinegar
6 clove of garlic, crushed through a press
Salt to taste

Combine ingredients (must be refrigerated first). Add drop by drop 5 tablespoons oil. Add lemon juice drop by drop as well. Add garlic and salt to taste. Whisk until well blended. Refrigerate until firm.

Chili Mayonnaise

1/2 cup mayonnaise
2 teaspoons chili powder
1 teaspoon ground cumin
2 teaspoons fresh lemon juice or vinegar
Dash salt
1/8 teaspoon cayenne pepper

In a small bowl, combine ingredients, except mayonnaise. Stir until well blended. Blend in mayonnaise.

(*) *The quantity alters for 4 egg yolks, by 8 tablespoons olive oil, lemon juice, salt, and 5 tablespoons water. There is some danger of salmonella from uncooked egg yolks.*

French Spicy Mayonnaise

1 cup mayonnaise
1 hard-boiled egg yolk, mashed
1 tablespoon chopped anchovies
1 tablespoon chopped parsley
1 tablespoon drained capers
1 teaspoon mustard
Dash cayenne pepper

In a small bowl, combine all ingredients. Stir until well blended. Cover and refrigerate.

Oriental Curry-Lemon Mayonnaise

1/2 cup mayonnaise
1/2 cup sour cream
1 1/2 teaspoons curry powder
1 tablespoon fresh lemon juice or vinegar
Dash salt
Dash cayenne pepper

1. In a small bowl, combine mayonnaise and sour cream. Mix until well blended. Stir in lemon juice, salt, and cayenne. Add curry powder.
2. Cover and refrigerate.

Creamy Avocado Dressing

1 avocado
1 clove garlic, crushed through a press
2 teaspoons olive oil
1/4 cup water
2 tablespoons sour cream
1 tablespoon fresh (or dried) dill
1/2 teaspoon sea salt
2 tablespoons lemon juice (or vinegar)

1. Peel avocado. Cut into large quarters.
2. In food processor, place ingredients. Process until creamy.

Dill Dip

1/2 cup mayonnaise
1/2 cup sour cream
2 tablespoons minced fresh dill (or 1 tablespoon dried dill)
2 tablespoons chopped parsley
2 tablespoons chopped scallions
1/2 teaspoon lemon juice or vinegar
1/2 teaspoon salt
1/2 teaspoon black pepper

In a small bowl, combine all ingredients. Stir until well blended. Refrigerate.

Cream Cheese Dip

2 8-ounce packages cream cheese, softened
1 scallion, minced
1 large clove garlic, crushed through a press
1 dash cayenne pepper
1 dash salt
1 dash vinegar or lemon juice
1/2 teaspoon dried dill
1/2 teaspoon dried basil
1/2 teaspoon dried marjoram
1/2 teaspoon dried thyme
1/2 teaspoon dried tarragon

> In a medium bowl, combine all ingredients. Stir until well blended. Cover and refrigerate.

Chutney Cheese Spread

1 8-ounce package cream cheese
2 cups shredded sharp Cheddar cheese (about 8 ounces)
2 tablespoons dry sherry
1/2 cup mango chutney, chopped
1/4 cup scallions, chopped
1 teaspoon curry powder
1/4 teaspoon salt
Dash hot pepper sauce or cayenne pepper

> In a medium bowl combine cream cheese, Cheddar cheese, curry powder, salt, hot sauce, and sherry. Blend until smooth and well blended. Cover and refrigerate until firm, about 2 hours. Top with chutney and sprinkle with scallions.

Horseradish Sauce

1 cup sour cream
1/3 cup horseradish
1 tablespoon fresh lemon juice or vinegar
Pinch white pepper

In a small bowl, combine all ingredients. Stir until well blended.
Cover and refrigerate 1 hour.

Blue Cheese Dip

1 cup blue cheese (4 ounces)
1 tablespoon white vinegar
1 scallion, chopped
1/2 cup mayonnaise
1/2 cup sour cream
1 clove garlic, crushed through a press

In a small bowl, combine all ingredients. Stir until well blended.
Cover and refrigerate.

NOTES

1. William Howard Hay: *A New Health Era*, Pocono Haven Publishing, 1933–1936.
2. IBID, page 140.
3. *NBC News*, January 6, 1997
4. Ragnar Berg: *Wholesome Food Nutrition for Mother and Child*, 5. Edition, Humata, 1986.
5. Friedrich F. Sander: *The Acid-Base Household of Human Organism*, Hippokrates, 1999.
6. Eduard Brecht: *Your Nutrition Is Your Destiny*, 6. Edition, Gewuerzmuehle, 1986.
7. Herman Aihara: *Basic Macrobiotics*, et al., Mahajiva Publishing, 1998.
8. B. Brenner: *Dietary Protein Intake and the Progressive Nature of Kidney Disease*, The New England Journal of Medicine 307, 632—No. 11, 1982.
9. Richard G. Klein: *The Human Career, Human Biological and Cultural Origins*, The University of Chicago Press, 1989.
10. Julian Jaynes: *The Origin of Consciousness in the Breakdown of the Bicameral Mind*, Houghton Mifflin, 1990.
11. American Diabetes Association.
12. CNN News, June 3, 1997.
13. Quazi S. Al Tariq, M.D., Horton Hospital (affiliate of New York Presbyterian Hospital), Arden Hill Hospital, Mid-Hudson Forensic Psych. Center, Goshen Residential Center.
14. IBID, Hay p. 42.
15. IBID, Tariq.
16. IBID, Tariq.
17. IBID, Tariq.
18. IBID, Tariq.
19. IBID, F.F. Sander.
20. IBID, Tariq.
21. CNN, *Headline News*, November 1996.
22. Hans Hermann Joergensen: *The Happy Molecule. Introduction into The Biochemistry of Minerals*; *with the Buffer-Capacity Raises and Falls Energy*, Medical Science, 6/93, 1988; *Acid-Alkaline Household—a Praxis-Near Procedure to Determine the Buffer-Capacity*, 5/2/1985, pp. 372–377 Medical Journal for Empirical Medical Science.
23. Eric Abraham Forsgren: *About the Rhythm of Liver-functions, Metabolism and Sleep*, Gumpert Publishing Gothenburg/Sweden.

24. Hilka de Groot-Boehlhoff, Professor Jutta Farhadi: *Issue of Nutrition,* Europe Textbook, 1989.
25. IBID, Groot-Boehlhoff, Farhadi.
26. American Heart Association, September 1998.
27. Claus Leitzmann, Professor of Nutrition, Justus Liebig University, Giessen.
28. American Dietetic Association, Publication: *A Primer on Fats and Oils.*
29. IBID, Groot-Boehlhoff, Farhadi.
30. Kilmar McCullym: *Homocysteine Revolution,* Group West, 1997.
31. *The Handy Science Answer Book,* p. 298, Visible Ink, 1994; Webster's New World Encyclopedia, p. 243; IBID, Groot-Boehlhoff, p. 63.
32. Judy Lin Eftekhar: *Feed Yourself Right*, Globe Communications, 1997, p. 43.
33. IBID, Groot-Boehlhoff, p. 128.
34. Professor Dr. Helmut Minne, M.D. (internal medicine) University Heidelberg; Chairman of the Board of Directors of the Kuratorium Knochengesundheit, e.v. (Kuratorium bone-health); Medical Director at Clinic The Fuerstenhof, Bad Pyrmont.
35. IBID, Eftekhar, p. 33.
36. *Webster's New World Encyclopedia,* p. 743.
37. *NBC Extra,* August 4, 1997.
38. IBID, Groot-Boehlhoff.
39. IBID, Eftekhar, p. 11.
40. Osteoporosis Foundation, CNN, January 9, 1997.
41. IBID, Hay.
42. IBID, Hay.
43. Good Housekeeping, July 1996, p. 104
44. IBID, Groot-Boehlhoff, p. 230
45. Webster's New World Encyclopedia, pp. 202, 203.

BIBLIOGRAPHY

Aihara, Herman.
—*Basic Macrobiotics,* 1998.
—*Acid and Alkaline,* by Herman Aihara, Stan Hodson, 1986.
Milk, a Myth of Civilization, by Herman Aihara, Jacques De Langre Aihara, 1984.

Berg, Ragnar.
—*Wholesome Food Nutrition for Mother and Child,* Humata, 1986.
—*Dictionary of Foods,* Gaylord Hauser, Ragnar Berg, Benedict Lust Publications, 2002.

Brecht, Eduard. *Your Nutrition Is Your Destiny,* Gewuerzmuehle, 1986.

Brenner, B. *Dietary Protein Intake and the Progressive Nature of Kidney Disease,* New England Journal of Medicine 307, 632—No.11, 1982.

De Groot-Boehlhoff, Hilka, Professor Farhadi, Jutta.
—*The Issue of Nutrition,* Europe Textbook, Nourney, Vollmer Publishing, Europa NrL. 60312, 1989.

Forsgren, Eric Abraham, *About the Rhythm of Liver-Functions, Metabolism and Sleep,* Bocktruckerie Aktiebolag, Stockholm, Verlag I Marcus, 1935.

Jaynes, Julian. *The Origin of Consciousness in the Breakdown of the Bicameral Mind,* Houghton Mifflin, 1990.

Joergensen, Hans Hermann.
—*The Happy Molecule: Introduction into the Biochemistry of Minerals.*

—With the Buffer Capacity Raises and Falls Energy, Medical Science, 6/93/1988.
—Acid-Alkaline Household—a Praxis-Near Procedure to Determine the Buffer Capacity, Medical Journal for Empirical Medical Science.

Klein, Richard. *The Human Career, Human Biological and Cultural Origins,* The University of Chicago Press, 1989.

Leitzmann, Claus.
—Dictionary of Nutrition/English/French/German/Italian/Spanish, Ulmer, 1996.
—Leitzmann, Claus, and Ibrahim Elmadfa: Nutrition of Humans, Ulmer 1999.
—Leitzmann, Claus, P. Glasauer, and J. Friedrich-Kaiser: Nutritional Help in Form of Milkproducts, Weltforum Publishing 1986.
—Leitzmann, Claus, Markus Keller, and Andreas Hahn: Alternative Nutrition, Hippokrates 1999.
—Leitzmann, Claus, Maria Weiger, and M. Kurz: Nutrition [by] Cancer, Graefe and Unzer 1996.

Ludwig, Walb.
—Revolutionary Cognition in Health Management, Medical Weekly 51,1940.
—Rheumatic Problems of the Practitioner Once and Now, Empirical Medical Science, 457, 1956
—Prevention of Chemical Imbalances, Medicine Today 1/8/1959.
—Prophylaxis of Allergic Diseases, Medicine Today 11/61.
—Prophylaxis of Kidney Diseases, Empirical Medical Science, 10/1962.
—About the Influence of Meaningful Nutrition, Empirical Medical Science, 9/13/1964.

—The Separation Cost, Especially for Kidney Diseases, Diaitia 6/1967.
—The Elektroneural-Diagnostic and—Therapy After Croon and the Significance of Objective Measured Data of Dysfunctional Body Functions. Physical Medicine and Rehabilitation, 7/9/1968.
—Simple Dietetics for the Practitioner. Magazine for General Medicine, 44, 29, 1968, 1434 ff.
—About the Effect of Separation Cost on Diabetes, Physical Medicine and Rehabilitation, 14, 9, 1973.
—Electro Diagnostic in the Practice, Empirical Medical Science, 4/24/1975.
—Dieting in Heart Therapy, Physical Medicine and Rehabilitation, 8/17/1976.
—Lecture About Croon's Method, Physical Medicine, 6/18/1977.
—Discussion Contribution to the Subject: Many Diet Concepts—Which One Should the Physician Follow in the Practice? Physical Medicine 8/18/1977.
—Detoxification with Separation Cost, Physical Medicine 6/21/1980.
—Nutrition Therapy with Separation Cost, Physical Medicine, 4/25/1984.

McCully, Kilmar. *Homocysteine Revolution,* Group West, 1997.

Sander, Friedrich. *The Acid-Base Household of Human Organism,* Hippokrates, 1999.

Seidl, Achim.
—The Emptiness of Zen, Diederichs Publishing, 1992.
—The Bi-Yaen-Lu, Hanser 1988.
—Psychosophie, Hanser 1992.

APPENDIX I

Researcher Dr. Friedrich F. Sander concluded that all severe illnesses, including **cardiac infarction** and **stroke**, are accompanied by a latent acidosis—i.e., hidden over-acidification, as in **diabetes mellitus, rheumatism, arthritis, and others**. Sander proved that latent acidosis in the tissues prepares the foundation for many illnesses *(The Acid-Base Household of Human Organism,* Hippokrates Publishing, 1985).

A study on 30 **obese women with increased blood-insulin** valence (University Bloemfontein in South Africa) has been published in the *American Journal of Clinical Nutrition* in 1994, No. 60, pages 48–53 (Slabber, M. et al.: Effects of low-insulin-response, energy-restricted diet on weight loss and plasma insulin concentrations in hyperinsulinemic obese females).

In a clinical scientific study on **diabetics** in 1980s, Dr. Ludwig Walb showed that after four to six weeks urine sugar measurements were reduced by 98% and the blood sugar measurements by 90%. The insulin-units could be reduced by 37%. The blood circulation improved. In five of his test subjects, the amputation of toes, foot, or lower leg could be avoided.

In a clinical scientific study in 1980, Dr. Ludwig Walb studied 620 patients from different disease groups. The serum **cholesterol** normalized within four weeks after changing to scientific eating in 86% of the cases.

In a clinical scientific study in 1978, Dr. Ludwig Walb studied 82 female and 51 male patients with an average of 58 years. The patients suffered from several illnesses, such as **disease of the heart and blood circulation** and the digestion organs, **diabetes, kidney diseases, rheum, tumors,** and **allergies**. The examined laboratory values improved by 80% in these four weeks. Particularly, the test was about following measurement sizes: white blood cells, calcium, Gamma GT, GPT and GOT, AP, erythrocyte sedimentation rate, uric acid, creatinin, urea nitrogen and urea, the proteins, as well as different blood fats, triglyceride, and entire cholesterol.

ical scientific study in 1990, Dr. Walb proved that scientific
uces coagulation clotting (measured by the "quick-value").

He proved in the laboratory that the quick-value for coagulation was lowered by scientific eating for 80% of his test persons. The recovery had been so successful because the blood became less viscous, which in turn reduced the risk of **cardiac infarction, thrombosis, and stroke**. Test persons with **heart and circulatory** problems were urged to avoid denatured food but instead were told to eat several smaller portions during the day. These test persons reported immediate relief.

In a clinical scientific study in 1984, Dr. Walb proved that over 90% of patients with high blood **cholesterol** levels reduced those levels after only four weeks of scientific eating; the origin of **arteriosclerosis** and its consequences, the calcification of coronary artery vessels and the burden of the circulation of blood, was essentially reduced.

Dr. Kilmer McCully linked in his research **homocysteine** to vitamin B deficiency. His findings were published in 1997.

In a clinical scientific study on 120 test persons who suffered from incurable kidney disease, Dr. Walb proved that higher levels of fluid excretion provide relief for the **heart and kidneys;** 80% of those incurable patients recovered or at least improved.

The Russian Nobel Prize recipient Ivan Pavlov performed experiments on dogs. Minced (cooked) meat fed to the dogs, was digested within approximately four hours. (Carbo-hydrates required 1.5 hours, or less.) But when Pavlov fed cooked meat and carbohydrates together to the dogs, their digestion was delayed considerably. Instead of the approximately four hours that the dogs usually needed for digesting the cooked meat, it took eight hours or longer for this incompatible food to pass through their stomachs to the duodenum and small intestines.

Researcher Dr. Berthold Kern concluded that cardiac infarctions and strokes are "acid-catastrophes."

In a clinical scientific study, Dr. Seyle and a team of Swiss researchers concluded that arteriosclerosis, condensed and altered vascular side, will improve or even normalize by eating according to scientific eating.

412

Furthermore, he pointed out that all serious illnesses such as diabetes mellitus, rheumatism, and arthritis, are accompanied by a latent acidosis.

Researcher Dr. Krone of the Max Planck Institute in Germany proved that the metabolism of cells could be altered in a positive sense as well as a negative sense through food.

APPENDIX II

A Big Piece Of The BioChemical Machine Puzzle
Some Background On Enzymes

Enzymes are biological catalysts capable of speeding up the chemical reactions necessary for life. However, regardless of what diet gurus say, enzymes do not possess magical properties that allow them to transcend the laws of body chemistry and "burn up calories before they hit your hips."[43]

In the last 30 years, as hundreds of enzymes have been identified in laboratory settings, it was believed that for every food there was an enzyme that would completely digest it, regardless of incompatible eating habits.

It's true that each chemical reaction in digestion requires its own particular enzyme. Digestive enzymes include amylase, which digests starch, lipase, which digests fats, and protease, which includes pepsin and is responsible for digesting proteins. Other enzymes play a part in the conversion of food energy into ATP (adenosine triphosphate), the power source for all cells in the body.

BUT, and here is the BIG BUT, for enzymes to reach their full effectiveness they require certain conditions, such as the right temperature, pH level, the availability of water, the right concentration, and the absence *of obstructive matter*. Temperature above 140°F/60°C damages (denatures) the intricate structure of enzymes, causing reactions to cease. Also, each enzyme operates best within a specific pH range and is denatured by *excessive acidity*. Acidity will prevent enzymes from speeding up the chemical reactions necessary for life. [44]

As you know, the A&B principles are all about avoiding excessive acidity, or the "obstructive matter" which reduces the effectiveness of enzymes.

The key to enzymes is to create an environment with a specific pH level that will allow them to operate effectively. By eating according to the A&B Method *the enzymes amylase and pepsin* will not be able *to hinder each other.*

Let's go back to our discussion of digestion, the switchboard of our very existence. According to *The World Book Encyclopedia:*

The digestive system consists primarily of the alimentary canal. As food moves through this canal, it is ground and mixed with various digestive juices. Most of these juices contain **digestive enzymes, chemicals that speed up reactions involved in the breakdown of food.** *When digestion is completed, starches and complex sugars are broken down into simple sugars; fats are digested to fatty acids and glycerol, and proteins are digested to amino acids and peptides. Simple sugars, fatty acids, glycerol, amino acids and peptides are the digested foods that can be absorbed into the bloodstream. The digestive juice in the stomach is called gastric juice. It contains hydrochloric acid and the enzyme pepsin. This juice begins the digestion of protein foods-starches, sugars, and fats are not digested by the gastric juice.* [45]

Why can't starches like bread be digested by the same gastric juice your body employs to break down cooked meat, cooked eggs and homogenized/pasteurized milk? Because the stomach is too acidic—the enzyme amylase that is necessary to break down starches can't possibly work. It loses its effectiveness when mixed with pepsin.

What happens to carbohydrates (starches, sugars), since they are *not* digested by the same gastric juice that breaks down proteins? Remember, carbohydrate digestion is different from acid-building protein digestion. A very important step in carbohydrate digestion occurs in the mouth. As you chew, the digestive enzyme amylase found in the saliva begins to split the starches and sugars into lower forms, preparing it for further reduction in the small intestine. Amylase acts best in an environment of positive alkalinity. Without an alkaline base there is no action of amylase on carbohydrate-rich foods. The slightest acid reaction slows down the splitting process and finally arrests this process of starchy reduction—*the food will not be completely digested.*

Also from *The World Book Encyclopedia:*

In the small intestine, the digestive process is completed on the partially digested food by pancreatic juice, intestinal juice, and bile. The pancreatic juice is produced by the pancreas and pours into the small intestine through a tube, or duct. The pancreatic juice contains the enzymes trypsin, amylase, and lipase. Trypsin breaks down the partly digested proteins, amylase changes starch into simple sugars, and lipase splits fats into fatty acids and glycerol. **When the food is completely digested,** *it is absorbed by tiny blood and lymph vessels in the walls of the small intestine. It is then carried by the bloodstream, throughout the body. Food particles are small enough to pass through the walls of the intestine and blood vessels—but only when they are completely digested.*[45]

If you don't eat according to your body chemistry by following the A&B Method, you will be unable to completely digest your food. None of the intestinal enzymes will function optimally in anything less than a positive alkaline medium. The alkaline state is maintained from the small intestine to the colon, or we could not digest our foods in the small intestine. If you eat incompatible mixtures of food, you create acidity that hinders the activity of your enzymes. Saliva, with its amylase, initiates starch digestion, *only* if the medium is alkaline, not otherwise. The gastric juice, with its pepsin, initiates protein digestion *only* if the medium is acid, not otherwise. The laws of your body chemistry are non-negotiable.

BioChemical Fact: Excessive acidity is the corpus delicti for most of our health and weight problems. When we eat in a chemically incompatible way, we hinder the enzymes from "speeding up" their chemical reactions, which slows down the metabolism. This, in turn, is the reason we get fat, fatigued, and ill.

Truth never dies. And the truth is that the enzyme amylase can't be optimally effective without an alkaline base and the enzyme pepsin can't be optimally effective if disturbed by amylase.

Enzymes work best in a specific pH range and are hindered or even denatured by excessive acidity and alkalinity. But your body will create no problem for you *when the food is completely digested.*

Acid-building ("bad" and "extreme bad") protein digestion is different from Neutral protein and carbohydrate digestion.

If you ignore this fact then you are demanding too much from your buffer system. Plainly put, you have to make sure that your foods are completely digested, so that no acidity will denature your enzymes. In this case, perhaps even the diet guru I mentioned before would be able to live up to her promise that *you burn up calories before they hit your hips.*[43]

APPENDIX III

Dr. William Howard Hay graduated from New York University on March 26, 1891, and practiced medicine and general surgery. After 16 years of practice devoted largely to general surgery, Dr. Hay came down with Bright's disease, an "incurable" kidney disease, accompanied by high blood pressure and a dilated heart. He received opiates and conventional treatment. Nothing helped, and he didn't recover. "There is no relief in medicine, but temporary relief," Dr. Hay said. It was this illness that changed Dr. Hay's view about medicine and surgery forever.

It was this key experience that led to his revolutionary discovery. He remembered an old report of a colonel in the British Army Medical Service, Robert McCarrison, who documented his observations and conclusions about the eating habits of the native people in India. Dr. Hay had nothing to lose. Immediately, he began eating like the native Himalayans.

Dr. Hay's medical problems slipped away. At the end of three months, he was again able to run long distances without distress. His weight dropped from 225 to 175 pounds. Years seemed to fall away, and he felt younger and stronger than he had in a long time. "It required a personal breakdown and a hopeless outlook for the future to really open [my] eyes to the possibilities of relief from disease along entirely different lines, however unorthodox these at first seemed," he said.

Based on his experiences and observations of the Himalayan's diet, Hays came to the conclusion that "all forms of disease and weight problems fall under one head—chemical imbalances of the body—and all are subject to restoration to the normal through correction of the body chemistry."

Dr. Hay closed his practice and founded his research institute in Pennsylvania where he dedicated 15 years to performing clinical research to develop and prove his theories about the acid-alkaline balance and the vital alkaline reserve. He started to publish his work which received a highly gratifying response. "The few thousands who have already benefited by resident treatment are but small in comparison to the thousands who have benefited through reading of the methods or studying and following the home course of management. The letters of thankfulness and appreciation received daily from so many who are complete strangers testify to the fact that the methods are so simple and effective that they can be successfully applied at any distance from personal supervision," he said.

INDEX